FNA Cytology of Ophthalmic Tumors

Monographs in Clinical Cytology

Vol. 21

Series Editor

Philippe Vielh Villejuif

FNA Cytology of Ophthalmic Tumors

Volume Editors

Charles V. Biscotti Cleveland, Ohio
Arun D. Singh Cleveland, Ohio

83 figures, 81 in color, and 6 tables, 2012

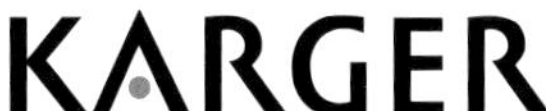

Basel · Freiburg · Paris · London · New York · New Delhi · Bangkok · Beijing · Tokyo · Kuala Lumpur · Singapore · Sydney

Monographs in Clinical Cytology

Charles V. Biscotti, MD
Department of Anatomic Pathology
Cleveland Clinic Foundation
9500 Euclid Avenue
Cleveland, OH 44195 (USA)
E-Mail biscotc@ccf.org

Arun D. Singh, MD
Professor of Ophthalmology
Director, Department of Ophthalmic Oncology
Cole Eye Institute, Cleveland Clinic Foundation
9500 Euclid Avenue
Cleveland, OH 44195 (USA)
E-Mail singha@ccf.org

Library of Congress Cataloging-in-Publication Data

FNA cytology of ophthalmic tumors / volume editors, Charles V. Biscotti, Arun D. Singh.
p. ; cm. -- (Monographs in clinical cytology, ISSN 0077-0809 ; v. 21)
Includes bibliographical references and index.
ISBN 978-3-8055-9870-5 (hard cover : alk. paper) -- ISBN 978-3-8055-9871-2 (electronic version)
I. Biscotti, Charles V. II. Singh, Arun D. III. Series: Monographs in clinical cytology ; v. 21. 0077-0809
[DNLM: 1. Biopsy, Fine-Needle--methods. 2. Eye Neoplasms--pathology. 3. Eye Neoplasms--diagnosis. W1 MO567KF v.21 2012 / WW 149]

616.99'484--dc23

2011037061

Bibliographic Indices. This publication is listed in bibliographic services, including Current Contents®.

www.karger.com
Printed in Switzerland on acid-free and non-aging paper (ISO 9706) by Reinhardt Druck, Basel
ISSN 0077–0809
ISBN 978–3–8055–9870–5
e-ISBN 978–3–8055–9871–2

We dedicate this volume to our families
– Janet, Ellen, and Julie
– Anna, Nakul, and Rahul
Without your love and support this work could not have been completed.

Contents

Preface

Ophthalmic cytology has emerged as an accepted and valuable diagnostic subspecialty. Surprising to most cytologists, definitive ophthalmic cancer therapy rarely requires cellular or tissue diagnosis. Experienced ophthalmologists can directly visualize ocular tumors and make accurate diagnoses in most cases. This fact does not diminish the importance of ophthalmic cytology. Rather it emphasizes the importance of close collaboration between cytologists and ophthalmologists when evaluating those clinically ambiguous cases that require corroboration. Indeed, this monograph emerged from our collaboration and recognition that accurate diagnoses require the contributions of both the cytologist and the ophthalmologist. Further, we recognized the need for a definitive and comprehensive source for ophthalmic cytology integrated with clinical ophthalmology.

We are greatly indebted to our twelve co-authors for contributing their time and expertise. Each brings valuable experience and their perspective to the respective topics. We took great care, during the editorial process, to create a relatively uniform layout, avoid overlap, and create a consistent presentation. We are also indebted to our publisher S. Karger for recognizing the need for this monograph and entrusting us with this task. We thank Mr. Thomas Nold and Mr. Stefan Sessler for their outstanding efforts. Finally, the secretarial assistance of Ms Deborah Mitchell is also greatly appreciated.

Charles V. Biscotti, MD,
Department of Anatomic Pathology, Cleveland Clinic,
Cleveland, Ohio, USA

Arun D. Singh, MD,
Department of Ophthalmic Oncology, Cole Eye Institute,
Cleveland Clinic, Cleveland, Ohio, USA

Chapter 1

Biscotti CV, Singh AD (eds): FNA Cytology of Ophthalmic Tumors.
Monogr Clin Cytol. Basel, Karger 2012, vol 21, pp 1–9

History, Indications, Techniques and Limitations

Arun D. Singh[a] · David E. Pelayes[c] · Jennifer A. Brainard[b] · Charles V. Biscotti[b]

[a]Cole Eye Institute and [b]Department of Anatomic Pathology, Cleveland Clinic Foundation, Cleveland, Ohio, USA;
[c]Department of Ophthalmology, University of Buenos Aires, Buenos Aires, Argentina

Relatively little has been published in the cytology or ophthalmology literature about the role and accuracy of fine needle aspiration (FNA) in the diagnosis of ophthalmic tumors [1–4]. In this article we explore various aspects of intraocular tumor FNA including historical aspects, indications, contraindications, techniques and surgical instruments, complications, and the limitations of the ophthalmic FNA cytology. A brief but critical appraisal of the literature is also included.

History

Although relatively recently accepted in the evaluation of ophthalmic tumors, FNA has a long and well-documented past. The first report of needle aspiration can be found in the writings of Abulcasis (936–1013 AD) in a book entitled *The Method of Medicine,* the most influential text of medieval Arab medicine. Abulcasis advocated puncture of the thyroid gland with a hollow needle for therapeutic purposes. Since microscopes would not be invented until the 1830s, it is unclear how the material obtained was evaluated. In 1847, M. Kün, a professor of physiology in Strasbourg, France, was the first to report use of a needle technique to obtain material for microscopy [5, 6]. Over the next 20–30 years, there were scattered reports of needle aspiration for diagnostic purposes. Only a minority of these reports focused on the diagnosis of potential malignancy. Most centered on the use of aspiration techniques to confirm infectious disease. In 1883, Leyden performed the first transthoracic needle aspiration of lung tissue to identify pneumonic organisms. In 1904, Grieg and Gray, British military surgeons, used a syringe and needle to aspirate liquid from the enlarged cervical lymph nodes of sleeping sickness sufferers to identify the motile trypanosomes [6, 7]. Soon thereafter, there were multiple reports of use of similar techniques to puncture lymph nodes for the diagnosis of secondary syphilis and leishmaniasis.

In 1870–1880, tissue stains were developed and mechanical microtomes were improved to the point where it became possible to prepare well-stained, thin tissue sections in a rapid and reliable manner [6, 8]. Tissue sections for pathological diagnosis quickly became the most widely accepted method for evaluating tumors and, by mid 1890, eclipsed early tissue cytology. In the first quarter of the 20th century, controversy raged over the diagnosis of cancer by means of aspirate smears rather than tissue sections. As a consequence, needle aspiration received little acceptance. The exception to this was the Memorial Hospital for Cancer and Allied Diseases in New York City (the present-day Memorial Sloan Kettering Cancer Center), where aspiration biopsy developed and flourished over a 30-year period as a result of a difference of opinion between a surgeon and the chief of pathology. Hayes E. Martin, a young head and neck surgeon, was at odds with James Ewing, chief of pathology, insisting that tissue diagnosis was required to advise and manage his patients appropriately. Ewing opposed open surgical biopsy believing that such procedures spread malignancy [9, 10]. A compromise was reached, and Martin began performing needle biopsies on a variety of neoplasms using 18-gauge needles. Martin worked closely with Edward Ellis, chief histotechnologist, and Fred Stewart, surgical pathologist, who prepared and interpreted smears and cell blocks. Eventually virtually every organ was sampled with the biopsy needle at Memorial Hospital [9]. In 1933, Stewart summarized the group's experience with 2,500 tumors analyzed by needle aspiration. Needle aspiration prospered at Memorial Hospital during the 30-year collaboration of Martin, Ellis and Stewart, but limited interest was shown by other centers in the USA. By the 1960s, with the increasing use of open biopsy, the technique was all but obsolete, even at Memorial Hospital.

Detractors of needle aspiration based their arguments on their belief that the technique was inherently inaccurate due to the small amount of material obtained. There was also a lack of trained personnel and standardized diagnostic criteria for cytology samples. Others feared the possibility of tumor seeding and spreading following the procedure. While these arguments were on the forefront in the USA, needle aspiration was undergoing resurgence in Europe. This may have arisen out of necessity. There was a severe shortage of pathologists in Europe after World War II, rendering accurate and timely pathological tissue diagnosis impossible. In the mid 1950s, Soderstrom and Franzen in Switzerland and Lopes-Cardozo in Holland, all hematologists by training, became major proponents and studied thousands of cases each year. These cytologist-clinicians popularized this technique using 22- and higher-gauge needles, with an external diameter of 6 mm or less [9]. These needles are termed 'fine needles'. Zajicek, Franzen and Lowhagen at the Karolinska Radiumhemmet Hospital in Sweden applied rigorous scientific methods to define diagnostic criteria in a variety of conditions. They emphasized the simplicity, safety, rapidity and diagnostic accuracy of the technique by presenting their findings with full clinical, histological and follow-up data [9]. Their contribution was immense in teaching others FNA and in influencing clinicians to adopt FNA as a diagnostic method. Use of this method has slowly increased over the years. Today in the USA, FNA enjoys selectively enthusiastic acceptance [9, 11, 12].

The first intraocular biopsy was performed by Hirschberg in 1868, and since then various surgical methods have been developed [2, 13–18]. FNA has only recently gained popularity for the diagnosis of orbital and intraocular tumors. In 1979, Jakobiec et al. [19] published a major report on the use of FNA for the diagnosis of intraocular tumors. Subsequently, ocular FNA has proven to be a generally safe and reliable means of obtaining diagnostic material [20–26].

The overwhelming majority of intraocular solid tumors can be diagnosed noninvasively, with clinical, angiographic and ultrasonographic studies obviating the need for diagnostic FNA. It is estimated that about 1–2% of cases will require diagnostic ocular FNA [24]. However, when indicated, ocular diagnostic FNA has proved to be effective with adequacy rates typically ranging from 88 to 95% [24, 27].

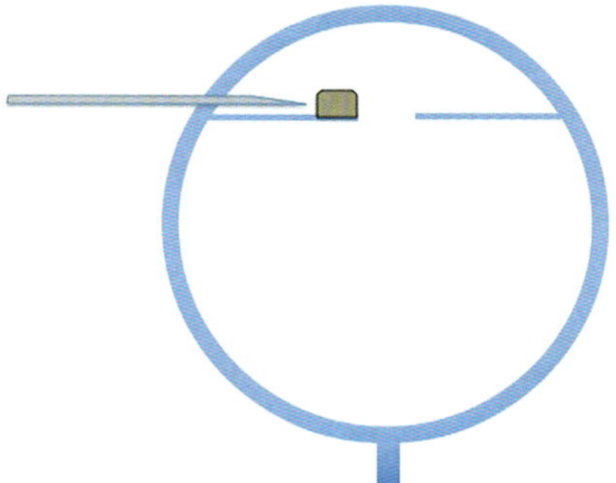

Fig. 1. Schematic representation of an FNAB of an iris tumor. Note that the needle bevel is up, the needle is parallel to the iris plane and the needle is not going across the pupil.

Techniques and Instrumentations

There are several techniques to obtain ocular biopsies for cytological or histopathological diagnosis including excisional biopsy, incisional biopsy, aspiration of ocular fluids (aqueous or vitreous) [28] and FNA biopsy (FNAB) [26, 29, 30]. The techniques for intraocular biopsy vary depending upon the involved tissue (retina, choroid, subretinal space, vitreous) [31, 32], suspected diagnosis, size, location, associated retinal detachment and clarity of the media [30, 33–36]. Although the present review is limited to FNAB, a brief mention of other techniques is also included.

Iris Tumors

In the case of iris tumors, the entry is through the anterior chamber (fig. 1) [37]. A 26- to 30-gauge needle is inserted at the slitlamp or in the operating room, at a 45- to 90-degree angle to the tumor. Gentle aspiration is performed while the needle is swept over the surface of the lesion aspirating about 0.5 ml of the aqueous humor [37]. Other authors have favored direct insertion of the needle into the tumor so as to maximize cellular yield even in a very cohesive tumor [38]. In patients suspected to have intraocular lymphoma with visible cells on biomicroscopy, anterior chamber paracentesis may be sufficient to yield the diagnosis [39]. Use of a 20-gauge [34] and 25-gauge vitrector has also been advocated for performing minimally invasive iridectomy yielding tissue for cytological and histopathological diagnosis

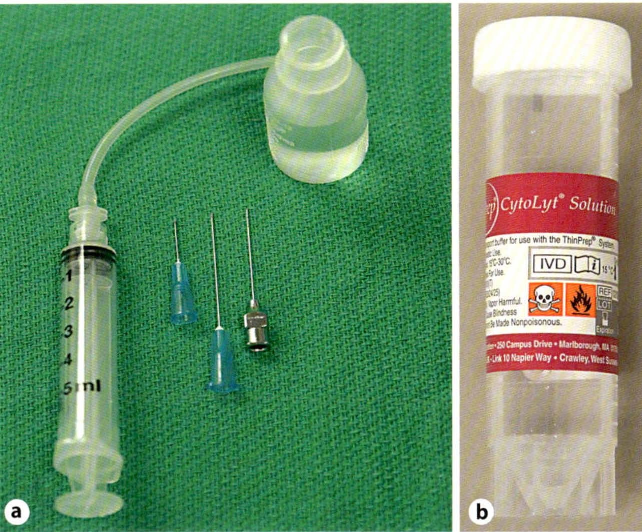

Fig. 2. A short 25-gauge needle attached to short tubing is inserted through the scleral bed into the tumor and aspiration is performed (**a**). The contents of the needle, tubing and syringe are then rinsed into a tube of Cytolyt or other suitable transport medium (**b**).

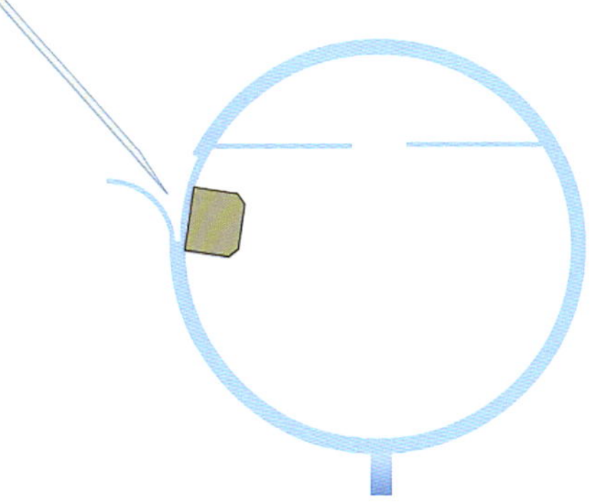

Fig. 3. Schematic representation of a transscleral FNAB of an anterior choroidal tumor. Note that the needle is inserted towards the center of the tumor under a partial thickness scleral flap.

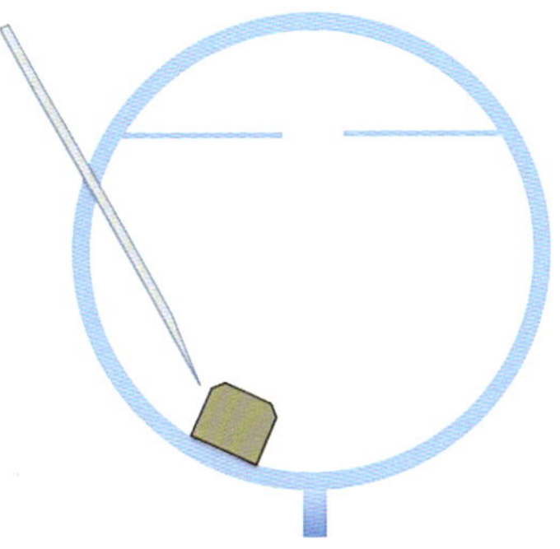

Fig. 4. Schematic representation of a transvitreal approach for FNAB of a posterior choroidal tumor. The entry point is 4 mm behind the limbus in the anteroposterior meridian of the tumor.

[40]. Overall, complications of iris biopsy such as persistent hyphema, prolonged hypotony, lens damage or endophthalmitis are extremely rare (<1%) [38].

Posterior Segment Tumors

Transscleral Approach

Tumors located in the ciliary body or anterior choroid can be biopsied transsclerally. A short 25-gauge needle attached to short tubing is needed (fig. 2). A 3-mm square scleral flap to a depth of approximately 80% is dissected. A small scratch-down incision is created in the scleral bed. The needle is then inserted through the scleral bed into the tumor and aspiration is performed (fig. 3). Posterior subretinal tumors with bullous retinal detachment may also be approached transsclerally using a tangential approach [24].

Transvitreal Approach

Posterior choroidal tumors are best accessible by a transvitreal approach (fig. 4). A 25- to 30-gauge needle, which is attached to a 5-ml syringe by a short tubing, is passed through the sclera into the vitreous 180° away at the pars plana 4 mm behind the limbus. The needle is advanced into the mid vitreous cavity and visualized through the pupil. Additional maneuvers are done either under indirect ophthalmoscopic control or a microscope depending upon the surgeon's preference [29]. Ultrasonic guidance is rarely used in the presence of clear media [19]. Once the needle tip has been inserted into the tumor avoiding major retinal or tumor vessels, gentle aspiration is performed by pulling the plunger up to the 2-ml mark. The needle can be either rotated along its long axis or moved in and out of the tumor minimally, so as to improve the cellular yield of the aspirate. Once the suction force has balanced out and without letting the plunger reset to its original position, the needle is withdrawn. Great care must be taken to make sure that the needle is withdrawn along the path of insertion [29]. Localized subretinal and/or vitreous hemorrhage is inevitable which is controlled by applying pressure to the globe by a cotton-tipped applicator at the entry site [29, 30, 41, 42]. If the globe softens, balanced salt solution can be injected into the vitreous cavity.

Needle Modifications

Most frequently used needles for ocular FNA are of 25–30 gauge (fig. 5). There is some evidence to suggest that the likelihood of insufficient samples may be lower with 22-gauge needles [41] and higher with 30-gauge needles [42]. All available 25- to 30-gauge needles have a bevel, which can limit full entry of the needle tip into a shallow tumor. Therefore, some authors have recommended bending the needle tip to 90° and entering the tumor tangentially rather than radially [29]. More recently, a prototype needle with a short bevel and millimeter graduations so as to improve awareness of the depth penetration has been evaluated (fig. 5) [43]. Preliminary data suggests that the aspirate with the prototype needle is more cellular than the standard 25-gauge needle [43].

Specific modifications of the tip of intraocular forceps allows it to retrieve tumor samples through retinotomy combined with 23-gauge 3-port vitrectomy (Essen forceps). The tumor sample is of sufficient size so as to allow histological and immunohistochemistry typing following cytoblock embedding [44].

Sample Handling

The contents of the needle, tubing and syringe are then rinsed into the tube of Cytolyt® or other suitable transport medium for processing, staining and cytological assessment of the sample [Chapter 2, this vol., pp. 10–16].

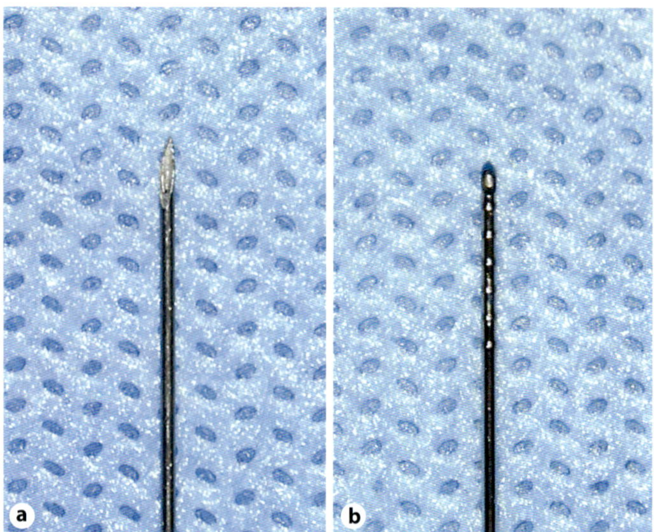

Fig. 5. A 25-gauge needle is most frequently used for ocular FNAB (**a**). Prototype graded needle with short bevel and surface millimeter markings (**b**).

Indications

There is some controversy regarding specific indications for intraocular FNAB [45]. In general, the major indication for FNA is when clinical examination and ancillary testing fail to establish an accurate diagnosis [24, 26, 46]. Potential scenarios include those with atypical clinical presentation, dense medium opacity, possible uveal metastasis without known primary tumor, and patients requesting histopathological confirmation before undergoing recommended therapy [29]. In our experience, ocular FNA is an effective technique to confirm a clinical diagnosis of malignancy including uveal metastasis [Chapter 3, this vol., pp. 17–30], uveal lymphoma [Chapter 4, this vol., pp. 31–43] or uveal melanoma [Chapter 5, this vol., pp. 44–54]. The clinical scenarios for uveal FNA include: confirm uveal metastasis, confirm uveal melanoma, melanoma versus metastasis, confirm uveal lymphoma, rule out metastasis, and rule out melanoma [22].

Amelanotic Uveal Tumor (Primary vs. Metastasis)

Uveal metastases are the most common uveal malignancy and approximately two thirds of uveal FNABs are performed to resolve a clinical differential diagnosis that includes metastasis and melanoma [Chapter 3, this vol., pp. 17–30] [24]. Shields et al. [24] have reported on the diagnostic effectiveness of intraocular FNA on 140 patients with intraocular malignancies such as uveal melanoma, uveal metastasis, retinoblastoma, lymphoma and leukemia. Histological correlation was available in 57 of cases, with histology-cytology diagnostic concordance in 54 of 57 (95%) cases. Augsburger et al. [22] examined 71 ocular FNA samples. Eleven of the 16 biopsies done to confirm a malignancy were for melanoma while 4 were for suspected metastases, 1 for suspected retinoblastoma and 1 for suspected medulloepithelioma. Histological correlation was available for 9 of those, and the cytological diagnoses were confirmed in 8 out of 9 cases. All 11 aspirates done to confirm benign conditions were read as benign [22].

Benign Pigmented Proliferations

Char et al. [47] performed intraoperative FNAB to diagnose benign pigmented proliferation such as melanocytoma, adenoma of the ciliary pigmented epithelium and retinal pigment epithelial hyperplasia prior to resection. There was complete agreement between the cytological and histopathological diagnoses in all 3 cases.

Nevus versus Melanoma (Indeterminate Melanocytic Lesions)

Transvitreal FNA with a 25-gauge needle has also been applied to differentiate between large choroidal nevus and small melanoma in patents with small melanocytic choroidal tumors (maximal diameter, ≤10 mm; thickness, 1.5–3.0 mm) [48]. A sufficient sample for diagnosis was obtained in only 22 of 34 cases (65%). Even so, tumors could not be classified as melanoma or nevus in 4 (12%, intermediate) cases. All 4 cases with intermediate lesions grew under observation and were treated as small melanoma. In addition 4 of the 12 tumors with insufficient samples were also subsequently reclassified as small choroidal melanomas on clinical grounds and treated. Two cases diagnosed cytologically as benign continued to remain stable [48]. Given that cellular yield is lower with smaller tumors [45, 49, 50] and even an expert cytopathologist may not be able to unequivocally distinguish a nevus from melanoma [26], we feel that such indeterminate melanocytic lesions (large nevus vs. small melanoma) should not be readily subjected to diagnostic FNA. Instead they should be managed by clinical criteria [51].

Melanoma: Diagnostic

In the case of intraocular melanoma [Chapter 5, this vol., pp. 44–54], a number of studies have shown that FNA has a diagnostic accuracy rate of over 90% [4, 24, 26, 46, 52]. Char et al. [53] observed FNA to be accurate in both the diagnosis and cytological typing of uveal melanomas. In their series, 26 of 29 (89%) tumors were accurately diagnosed, and 14 of 18 (78%) cases showed correlation of predominant cell types [53]. In their subsequent article, Char et al. [54] found FNA to be accurate in the diagnosis of all cases of iris ring melanoma. Czerniak et al. [20] found FNA to be diagnostically accurate and concluded that it could be used to establish the predominant cell type (spindle vs. epithelioid). Shields et al. [24] have also reported similar results, with 26 of 27 (96%) patients diagnosed on FNA to have uveal melanoma being subsequently proven to have melanoma on enucleation.

Melanoma: Prognostic

A further indication for uveal FNA is to perform prognostic studies for uveal melanoma [Chapter 6, this vol., pp. 55–60] [55].

Intraocular Lymphoma

Ocular FNA correctly identified the two patients in our series with primary uveal lymphoma [56]. Both uveal lymphoma specimens were cytologically consistent with uveal lymphoma. The role of FNA in the diagnosis of uveal lymphoma is discussed elsewhere [Chapter 4, this vol., pp. 31–43]. However, vitrectomy and not FNA is required to diagnose primary vitreoretinal lymphoma (ophthalmic variant of primary central nervous system lymphoma) as it predominantly manifests as lymphocytic infiltration of the vitreous [Chapter 7, this vol., pp. 61–71] [57]. Cellular assessment is often done in conjunction with ancillary studies, such as immunohistochemistry or flow cytometry [58, 59]. Even then, the sample may be insufficiently cellular for a definitive morphological diagnosis or ancillary studies [60].

Retinoblastoma and Other Retinal Tumors

FNAB is recommended only in highly selected cases of retinal tumors where there is a true diagnostic dilemma after all possible clinical investigations including an opinion by an expert ocular oncologist have been obtained [Chapter 8, this vol., pp. 72–81].

Orbital Tumors

The role of orbital FNAB particularly for lacrimal gland tumors, lymphoproliferative tumors and metastatic lesions of the orbit is discussed in Chapter 9 [this vol., pp. 82–89].

Contraindications

FNA is contraindicated in uveal masses with well-established diagnosis, small choroidal or iris melanocytic lesions in which the differential diagnosis is between a large nevus or small melanoma, and iris, ciliary body or choroidal mass with documented enlargement and planned resection [24]. The limited role of FNA in the setting of retinoblastoma is discussed in Chapter 8 [this vol., pp. 72–81].

Limitations

Insufficient Sample or False-Negative Biopsy

Limited cellularity can compromise the diagnostic potential of ocular aspirate samples [54]. In our series of 30 unpublished cases, 4 had limited cellularity. Two of the cases were signed out as 'atypical cells', 1 was read as 'negative' and 1 as 'nondiagnostic'. In both cases of 'atypical cells', we were able to suggest the correct underlying pathology (a metastatic carcinoid and a benign nevus). The patient whose biopsy was read as 'negative' subsequently underwent incisional biopsy which revealed a uveal schwannoma [61]. Perhaps the presence of a dispersed bland spindle cell composition in the schwannoma could explain the lack of a specific diagnosis by FNA. The second case, read as 'nondiagnostic', showed only histiocytes. Because of strong clinical suspicion of choroidal melanoma, enucleation done a week later revealed diffuse choroidal melanoma with changes secondary to prior treatment. The melanoma had been treated previously (inadvertently) with intravitreal injections of bevacizumab [62]. In their case series, Augsburger et al. [22] reported 2 false-negative cases out of 5 total negative reports.

Important practical considerations to reduce the likelihood of a nondiagnostic biopsy are summarized (table 1). It can be concluded that a negative cytological diagnosis of malignancy should not be considered unequivocal proof that an intraocular malignancy does not exist [22]. Others have also echoed similar views regarding unreliability of negative diagnoses [26, 45].

Incorrect or False-Positive Findings

The overall concordance between histological findings and cytological diagnosis (in experienced centers) may be as high as 95% [4, 22]. In particular, uveal melanocytomas can pose a diagnostic challenge [22]. One case of melanocytoma was diagnosed as melanoma but turned out to be melanocytoma on histology [22]. Faulkner-Jones et al. [63] reported a false-positive cytological diagnosis of malignancy in a patient with a ciliary body hemangioma.

Table 1. Practical considerations to reduce the likelihood of a non-diagnostic ocular FNAB

Factors	Guidance
Tumor size	avoid small tumors (less than 2.5 mm in height)
Needle size	avoid thinner needle (such as 30 gauge)
Aspiration	avoid plunger retraction once aspiration has been completed
Sample	avoid dry smears; rinse the needle into a transport medium flushing the contents of the needle and syringe several times
Experience	practice on enucleated globes to become familiarized with the techniques
Personnel	experienced cytopathologist is essential

These are personal recommendations. May vary between centers.

Complications

Needle Tract Seeding

One of the main reasons for failure of early adoption of FNA as a diagnostic tool was concern over the possibility of needle tract seeding of malignant cells and tumor dissemination. It is well known that, in general, the risk of complications associated with FNA decreases with the diameter of the needle. There have been at least 12 reports of needle tract seeding linked directly to the FNA procedure [64]. Local dissemination has also been reported but is exceedingly rare. Needle sizes associated with these reports were relatively large (19–21 gauge) or not reported. There have been no documented reports of local tumor extension caused by small diameter needles (23 gauge or higher). A study performed at the Karolinska Institute in Sweden followed 656 patients who underwent cervical lymph node FNA diagnostic of metastatic malignancy using 22-gauge needles. These patients were followed for 5 years, and no patient showed evidence of local tumor growth. Also, in experimental models [65] and in studies of survival rates of patients with breast cancer [66] and thyroid nodules [67], there were no differences noted between groups with and without FNA. Using thinner needles and releasing negative pressure before withdrawing the needle may further reduce the already miniscule risk of seeding. This has proven to be true in the ophthalmic FNA. The number of tumor cells in the scleral tracts of 30-gauge needles was lower when the needle transversed the aqueous or vitreous [68]. Even so, the number of cells was not enough to cause tumor growth in an experimental model [68]. In more than 200,000 cases of transocular FNA in the literature, there has been no evidence of local or systemic spread of tumor cells with the use of 25-gauge or smaller diameter needles [22, 24, 38, 46, 68–70].

Hemorrhage

The most frequent complications are localized subretinal and vitreous hemorrhage at the biopsy site [24, 29]. The hemorrhage is controlled by gentle pressure on the globe immediately after withdrawal of the needle. The hemorrhages typically clear within a few weeks (fig. 6).

Retinal Detachment

The retinal break created when a subretinal tumor is biopsied transvitreally almost never leads to rhegmatogenous retinal detachment. The break is sealed by the blood clot at the biopsy site (fig. 7).

Endophthalmitis

Only 2 cases of post-FNAB endophthalmitis have been reported [49, 63]. It is essential to perform ocular FNAB under sterile conditions.

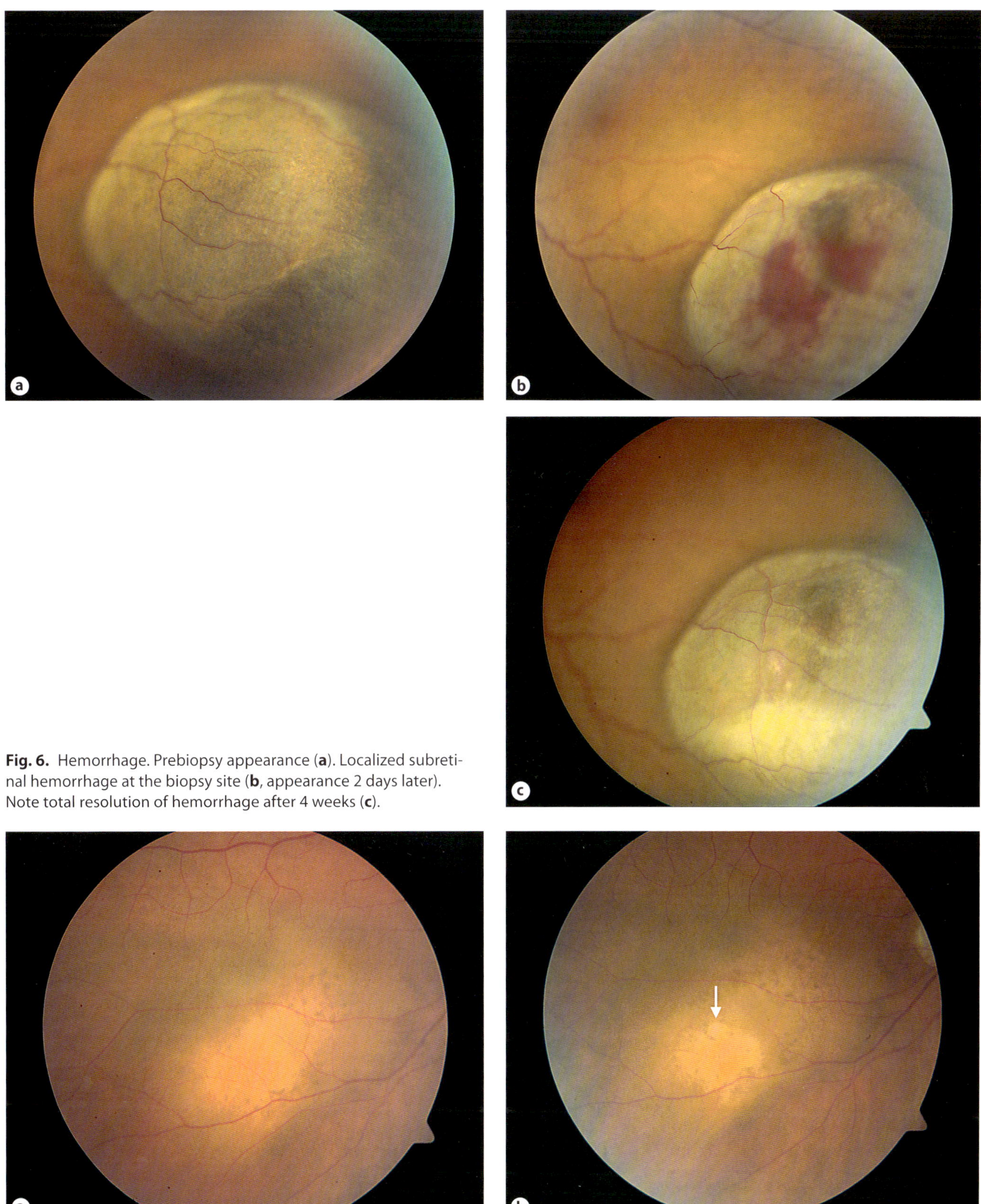

Fig. 6. Hemorrhage. Prebiopsy appearance (**a**). Localized subretinal hemorrhage at the biopsy site (**b**, appearance 2 days later). Note total resolution of hemorrhage after 4 weeks (**c**).

Fig. 7. Retinal detachment. Prebiopsy appearance (**a**). Spontaneous closure of the retinal break created during transvitreal FNAB (**b**, arrow).

Conclusions

The vast majority of uveal tumors can be diagnosed based on clinical examination and ocular imaging studies, which obviate the need for diagnostic ocular FNA. Overall, diagnostic accuracy of ocular FNA is high but limited cellularity can compromise the diagnostic potential of ocular aspirate samples. The role of ocular FNA is limited in retinal tumors. Orbital FNA should be considered in the evaluation of lacrimal gland tumors, orbital metastasis and lymphoproliferative lesions. Negative cytological diagnosis of malignancy should not be considered unequivocal proof that an intraocular malignancy does not exist. With improved understanding of genetic prognostic factors of uveal melanoma, ocular FNA is gaining popularity for prognostic purposes in combination with eye-conserving treatment of the primary tumor. In special clinical indications, ancillary studies such as immunohistochemistry and fluorescence in situ hybridization can be performed on ocular FNA samples. Assistance of an experienced cytopathologist cannot be overemphasized.

References

1 Sanders TE: Intraocular biopsy: an evaluation. Trans Am Ophthalmol Soc 1952;50:375–405.
2 Long JC, Black WC, Danielson RW: Aspiration biopsy in intraocular tumors. AMA Arch Ophthalmol 1953;50:303–310.
3 Andersen SR. Biopsy in intraocular tumours: a preliminary report. Acta Ophthalmol (Copenh) 1954;32:645–657.
4 Augsburger JJ: Fine needle aspiration biopsy of suspected metastatic cancers to the posterior uvea. Trans Am Ophthalmol Soc 1988;86:499–560.
5 Long SR, Cohen MB: Classics in cytology. VII. Kun, Lebert, and early efforts at fine-needle aspiration biopsy. Diagn Cytopathol 1996;14:182–183.
6 Webb AJ: Early microscopy: history of fine needle aspiration (FNA) with particular reference to goitres. Cytopathology 2001;12:1–6.
7 Ansari NA, Derias NW: Fine needle aspiration cytology. J Clin Pathol 1997;50:541–543.
8 Rosa M: Fine-needle aspiration biopsy: a historical overview. Diagn Cytopathol 2008;36:773–775.
9 Frable WJ: Fine-needle aspiration biopsy: a review. Hum Pathol 1983;14:9–28.
10 Hajdu SI, Ehya H. Foundation of diagnostic cytology. Ann Clin Lab Sci 2008;38:296–299.
11 Lang WR, Strigari LL: The history of the American Society of Cytology. Acta Cytologica 1977;21:608–615.
12 Kline TS, Neal HS: Needle aspiration biopsy: a critical appraisal. Eight years and 3,267 specimens later. JAMA 1978;239:36–39.
13 Veasey CA Jr: Intraocular biopsy. Am J Ophthalmol 1951;34:432–434.
14 Jensen OA, Andersen SR: Late complications of biopsy in intraocular tumors. Acta Ophthalmol (Copenh) 1959;37:568–575.
15 Takemura T, Tomatsu Y: Studies on malignant melanoma of the choroid. I. Needle biopsy, light microscopy, and electron microscopy (in Japanese). Nippon Ganka Gakkai Zasshi 1967;71:1317–1322.
16 Makley TA Jr: Biopsy of intraocular lesions. Am J Ophthalmol 1967;64(suppl):591–599.
17 Sagiroglu N, Ozgonul T, Muderris S: Diagnostic intraocular cytology. Acta Cytol 1975;19:32–37.
18 Grgic Z, Ljustina-Ivancic N: Cytomorphologic findings in the diagnosis of intraocular lymphocytic tumors (author's transl; in German). Klin Monatsbl Augenheilkd 1978;173:416–418.
19 Jakobiec FA, Coleman DJ, Chattock A, Smith M: Ultrasonically guided needle biopsy and cytologic diagnosis of solid intraocular tumors. Ophthalmology 1979;86:1662–1681.
20 Czerniak B, Woyke S, Domagala W, Krzysztolik Z: Fine needle aspiration cytology of intraocular malignant melanoma. Acta Cytol 1983;27:157–165.
21 Char DH, Miller TR: Fine needle biopsy in retinoblastoma. Am J Ophthalmol 1984;97:686–690.
22 Augsburger JJ, Shields JA, Folberg R, Lang W, O'Hara BJ, Claricci JD: Fine needle aspiration biopsy in the diagnosis of intraocular cancer: cytologic-histologic correlations. Ophthalmology 1985;92:39–49.
23 Midena E, Segato T, Piermarocchi S, Boccato P: Fine needle aspiration biopsy in ophthalmology. Surv Ophthalmol 1985;29:410–422.
24 Shields JA, Shields CL, Ehya H, Eagle RC Jr, De Potter P: Fine-needle aspiration biopsy of suspected intraocular tumors: the 1992 Urwick lecture. Ophthalmology 1993;100:1677–1684.
25 Eide N, Syrdalen P, Walaas L, Hagmar B: Fine needle aspiration biopsy in selecting treatment for inconclusive intraocular disease. Acta Ophthalmol Scand 1999;77:448–452.
26 Eide N, Walaas L: Fine-needle aspiration biopsy and other biopsies in suspected intraocular malignant disease: a review. Acta Ophthalmol 2009; 87:588–601.
27 Char DH, Miller T: Accuracy of presumed uveal melanoma diagnosis before alternative therapy. Br J Ophthalmol 1995;79:692–696.
28 Green WR: Diagnostic cytopathology of ocular fluid specimens. Ophthalmology 1984;91:726–749.
29 Augsburger JJ, Shields JA: Fine needle aspiration biopsy of solid intraocular tumors: indications, instrumentation and techniques. Ophthalmic Surg 1984;15:34–40.
30 Char DH: Intraocular biopsy; in Singh AD, Damato BE, Pe'er J, Murphree AL, Perry JD (eds): Clinical Ophthalmic Oncology. Philadelphia, Saunders-Elsevier, 2007, pp 334–340.
31 Fastenberg DM, Finger PT, Chess Q, Koizumi JH, Packer S: Vitrectomy retinotomy aspiration biopsy of choroidal tumors. Am J Ophthalmol 1990;110:361–365.
32 Arbour JD, Mukai S: Biopsy of the retina and the choroid. Int Ophthalmol Clin 1999;39:213–222.
33 Foulds WS: The uses and limitations of intraocular biopsy. Eye 1992;6:11–27.
34 Bechrakis NE, Foerster MH, Bornfeld N: Biopsy in indeterminate intraocular tumors. Ophthalmology 2002;109:235–242.
35 Kvanta A, Seregard S, Kopp ED, All-Ericsson C, Landau I, Berglin L: Choroidal biopsies for intraocular tumors of indeterminate origin. Am J Ophthalmol 2005;140:1002–1006.
36 Sen J, Groenewald C, Hiscott PS, Smith PA, Damato BE: Transretinal choroidal tumor biopsy with a 25-gauge vitrector. Ophthalmology 2006; 113:1028–1031.
37 Grossniklaus HE: Fine-needle aspiration biopsy of the iris. Arch Ophthalmol 1992;110:969–976.
38 Shields CL, Manquez ME, Ehya H, Mashayekhi A, Danzig CJ, Shields JA: Fine-needle aspiration biopsy of iris tumors in 100 consecutive cases: technique and complications. Ophthalmology 2006;113:2080–2086.
39 Finger PT, Papp C, Latkany P, Kurli M, Iacob CE: Anterior chamber paracentesis cytology (cytospin technique) for the diagnosis of intraocular lymphoma. Br J Ophthalmol 2006;90:690–692.
40 Finger PT, Latkany P, Kurli M, Iacob C: The Finger iridectomy technique: small incision biopsy of anterior segment tumours. Br J Ophthalmol 2005;89:946–949.
41 Shields JA, Shields CL, Ehya H, Eagle RC Jr, De Potter P: Fine-needle aspiration biopsy of suspected intraocular tumors. Int Ophthalmol Clin 1993;33:77–82.
42 Young TA, Burgess BL, Rao NP, Glasgow BJ, Straatsma BR: Transscleral fine-needle aspiration biopsy of macular choroidal melanoma. Am J Ophthalmol 2008;145:297–302.
43 Singh AD, Pelayes D, Zarate JO, Biscotti CV. FNAB of uveal melanoma with a graded prototype needle. ARVO Meet Abstr 2011;52:3270.

44 Akgul H, Otterbach F, Bornfeld N, Jurklies B: Intraocular biopsy using special forceps: a new instrument and refined surgical technique. Br J Ophthalmol 2011;95:79–82.
45 Seregard S: To biopsy or not to biopsy? Acta Ophthalmol 2009;87:586–587.
46 Pelayes DE, Zarate JO: Fine needle aspiration biopsy with liquid-based cytology and adjunct immunohistochemistry in intraocular melanocytic tumors. Eur J Ophthalmol 2010;20:1059–1065.
47 Char DH, Miller TR, Crawford JB: Cytopathologic diagnosis of benign lesions simulating choroidal melanomas. Trans Am Ophthalmol Soc 1991;89:235–244, discussion 245–250.
48 Augsburger JJ, Correa ZM, Schneider S, et al: Diagnostic transvitreal fine-needle aspiration biopsy of small melanocytic choroidal tumors in nevus versus melanoma category. Trans Am Ophthalmol Soc 2002;100:225–232, discussion 232–234.
49 Cohen VM, Dinakaran S, Parsons MA, Rennie IG: Transvitreal fine needle aspiration biopsy: the influence of intraocular lesion size on diagnostic biopsy result. Eye (Lond) 2001;15:143–147.
50 Shields CL, Ganguly A, Materin MA, et al: Chromosome 3 analysis of uveal melanoma using fine-needle aspiration biopsy at the time of plaque radiotherapy in 140 consecutive cases: the Deborah Iverson, MD, Lectureship. Arch Ophthalmol 2007;125:1017–1024.
51 Singh AD, Schachat AP, Diener-West M, Reynolds SM: Small choroidal melanoma. Ophthalmology 2008;115:2319–2319.
52 Davila RM, Miranda MC, Smith ME: Role of cytopathology in the diagnosis of ocular malignancies. Acta Cytol 1998;42:362–366.
53 Char DH, Miller TR, Ljung BM, Howes EL Jr, Stoloff A: Fine needle aspiration biopsy in uveal melanoma. Acta Cytol 1989;33:599–605.
54 Char DH, Kemlitz AE, Miller T, Crawford JB: Iris ring melanoma: fine needle biopsy. Br J Ophthalmol 2006;90:420–422.
55 Sisley K, Rennie IG, Parsons MA, et al: Abnormalities of chromosomes 3 and 8 in posterior uveal melanoma correlate with prognosis. Genes Chromosomes Cancer 1997;19:22–28.
56 Fuller ML, Sweetenham J, Schoenfield L, Singh AD: Uveal lymphoma: a variant of ocular adnexal lymphoma. Leuk Lymphoma 2008;49:2393–2397.
57 Char DH, Ljung BM, Deschenes J, Miller TR: Intraocular lymphoma: immunological and cytological analysis. Br J Ophthalmol 1988;72:905–911.
58 Davis JL, Solomon D, Nussenblatt RB, Palestine AG, Chan CC: Immunocytochemical staining of vitreous cells: indications, techniques, and results. Ophthalmology 1992;99:250–256.
59 Davis JL, Viciana AL, Ruiz P: Diagnosis of intraocular lymphoma by flow cytometry. Am J Ophthalmol 1997;124:362–372.
60 Farkas T, Harbour JW, Davila RM: Cytologic diagnosis of intraocular lymphoma in vitreous aspirates. Acta Cytol 2004;48:487–491.
61 Turell ME, Hayden BC, McMahon JT, Schoenfield LR, Singh AD: Uveal schwannoma surgery. Ophthalmology 2009;116:163–163.
62 Lima BR, Schoenfield LR, Singh AD: The impact of intravitreal bevacizumab therapy on choroidal melanoma. Am J Ophthalmol 2011;151:323–328.
63 Faulkner-Jones BE, Foster WJ, Harbour JW, Smith ME, Davila RM: Fine needle aspiration biopsy with adjunct immunohistochemistry in intraocular tumor management. Acta Cytol 2005;49:297–308.
64 Wu M, Burstein DE: Fine needle aspiration. Cancer Invest 2004;22:620–628.
65 Eriksson O, Hagmar B, Ryd W: Effects of fine-needle aspiration and other biopsy procedures on tumor dissemination in mice. Cancer 1984; 54:73–78.
66 Liebens F, Carly B, Cusumano P, et al: Breast cancer seeding associated with core needle biopsies: a systematic review. Maturitas 2009:113–123.
67 Polyzos SA, Anastasilakis AD: A systematic review of cases reporting needle tract seeding following thyroid fine needle biopsy. World J Surg 2010;34:844–851.
68 Glasgow BJ, Brown HH, Zargoza AM, Foos RY: Quantitation of tumor seeding from fine needle aspiration of ocular melanomas. Am J Ophthalmol 1988;105:538–546.
69 Karcioglu ZA, Gordon RA, Karcioglu GL: Tumor seeding in ocular fine needle aspiration biopsy. Ophthalmology 1985;92:1763–1767.
70 Char DH, Kemlitz AE, Miller T: Intraocular biopsy. Ophthalmol Clin North Am 2005;18:177–185.

Arun D. Singh, MD, Professor of Ophthalmology
Director, Department of Ophthalmic Oncology, Cole Eye Institute, Cleveland Clinic Foundation
9500 Euclid Avenue
Cleveland, OH 44195 (USA)
Tel. +1 216 445 9479, E-Mail singha@ccf.org

Biscotti CV, Singh AD (eds): FNA Cytology of Ophthalmic Tumors.
Monogr Clin Cytol. Basel, Karger 2012, vol 21, pp 10–16

Cytological Preparation

Jennifer A. Brainard · Charles V. Biscotti

Department of Anatomic Pathology, Cleveland Clinic Foundation, Cleveland, Ohio, USA

The fundamental principle of fine needle aspiration (FNA) is to obtain a satisfactory aspirate sample that provides a true reflection of the disease process in the patient, allowing therapeutic decision-making [1, 2]. In spite of a controversial beginning, this biopsy method, as it has been studied and refined over the years, has proven to be accurate, simple, safe, rapid and cost effective with few contraindications [2–4]. A mass anywhere in the body accessible by a fine needle can be evaluated by FNA. It is readily performed on superficial palpable masses, most commonly lymph nodes, breast, soft tissue and salivary glands. Advances in radiological techniques have allowed access to deep-seated, nonpalpable masses, generally with ultrasound or CT guidance, including the eye and ocular adnexa.

Smear Preparation

The technique of performing an FNA of the eye is discussed in Chapter 1 [this vol., pp. 1–9]. Once the aspirate is obtained, samples may be processed in a variety of ways. The method selected depends on the clinical setting, the characteristics of the aspirate sample, and the preferences of the ophthalmologist and cytopathologist. In general, aspirate smears, needle rinses and cell blocks, alone or in combination, are prepared from a given sample.

Aspirate Smears

A close attention to smearing technique is required to maximize the diagnostic yield if aspirate smears are preferred. As ocular aspirate samples may yield minimal material depending on the site, smear preparation that avoids introduction of artifacts is critical. The aspirate sample is expressed onto clean, appropriately labeled glass slides. A variety of smearing techniques may be employed. One common technique is placement of a drop of the aspirated material in the center of a glass slide. It is important that the needle is placed bevel side down and is touching the glass slide. This prevents introduction of air-drying artifacts. A second glass slide is inverted and placed directly on top of the first slide. As the drop of aspirate material starts to spread, the two slides are gently pulled in opposite directions in a single motion, producing 2 smears that have aspirated material covering a small area in the center of the slide (fig. 1) [3, 5].

An alternate technique is placement of a drop of aspirated material near the frosted end of a glass slide. A second slide, placed perpendicularly over the drop is used to gently spread the aspirate material down the center of the first slide (fig. 2). This results in preparation of a single slide, with minimal material on the 'spreader slide'. Regardless of smearing preference, care should be taken to apply gentle constant pressure on the slides to prevent crush artifact and uneven smear thickness. Smear preparation artifacts may render an otherwise cellular sample nondiagnostic (fig. 3).

Needle Rinse Samples

Needle rinse samples from an FNA are processed using one of several standard concentration methods. Traditional concentration methods include millipore filtration and cytospin preparation. Newer, liquid-based thin-layer processing methods including Thinprep® (Hologic Inc., Marlborough, Mass., USA) and BD Cytorich Systems® (BD, Franklin Lakes, N.J., USA) involve rinsing the needle in a proprietary preservative solution followed by automated processing.

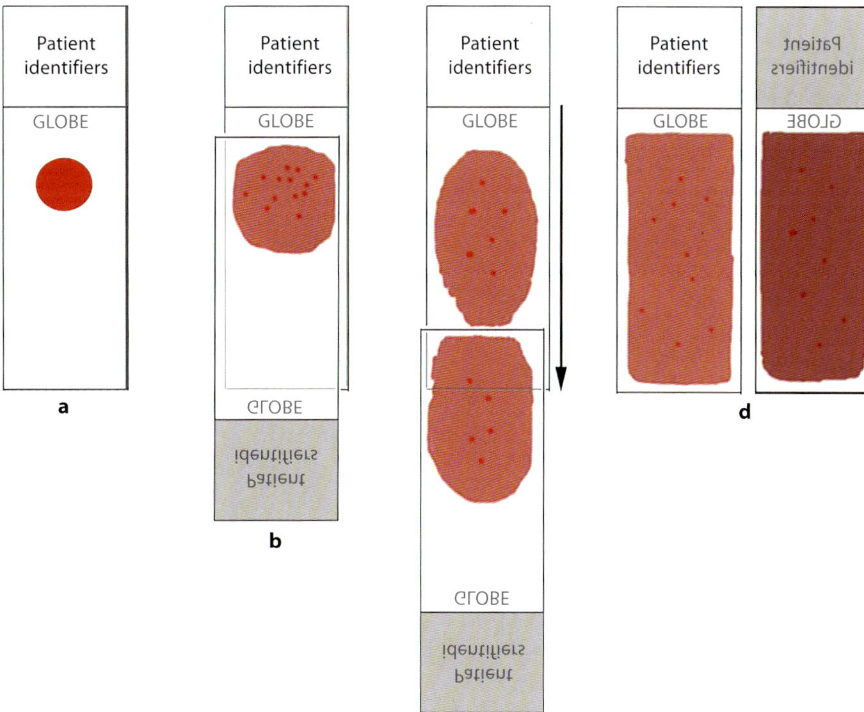

Fig. 1. A drop of sample is placed near the frosted end of a glass slide (**a**). A second slide is inverted over the sample, making gentle contact with the sample (**b**). The slides are pulled apart, maintaining even contact (**c**), resulting in 2 evenly covered slides with cellular material concentrated in the center (**d**). Courtesy Deborah Chute, MD.

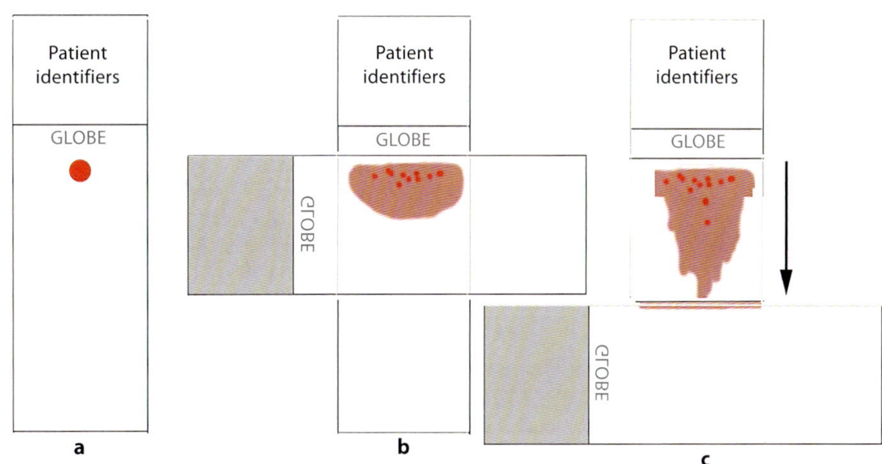

Fig. 2. A drop of sample is placed near the frosted end of a glass slide (**a**). A second slide is placed perpendicularly over the sample, making contact with the sample (**b**). The second slide is pulled down the first slide, maintaining even contact (**c**). The result is one slide with material concentrated in the center and one 'spreader' slide that may be discarded. Courtesy Deborah Chute, MD.

Both the Thinprep and BD Cytorich systems offer advantages over conventional cytospin and millipore filter preparations including standard processing, excellent cell preservation, a clean background and more even cellular dispersion with cells deposited in a thin layer, approaching a monolayer, in the center of the slide [6, 7]. Thus, artifacts including air drying, uneven cell dispersion, crush and excess blood are mitigated using these methods.

At our institution, we use the Thinprep processing system for nongynecological cytology specimens including ocular samples. In certain ocular FNA specimens, only one needle pass is possible or minimal aspirate material is anticipated. In these cases, we do not make aspirate smears, but place all material in Cytolyt® solution for Thinprep processing (fig. 4). The sample in Cytolyt is then subjected to one or more centrifugation and concentration steps. The pellet obtained

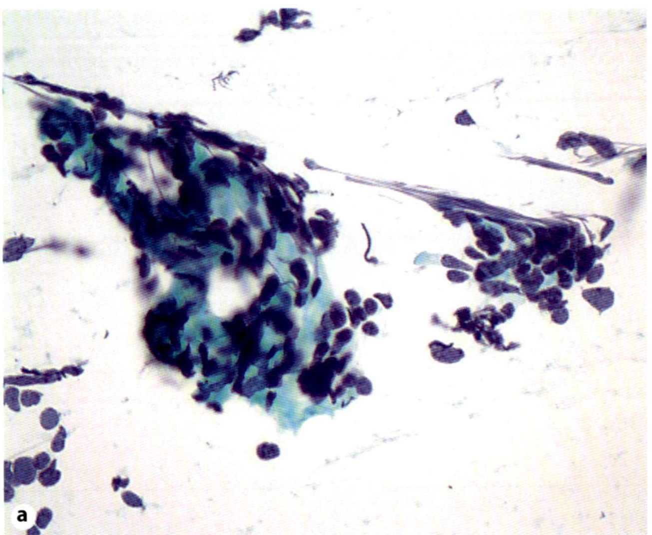

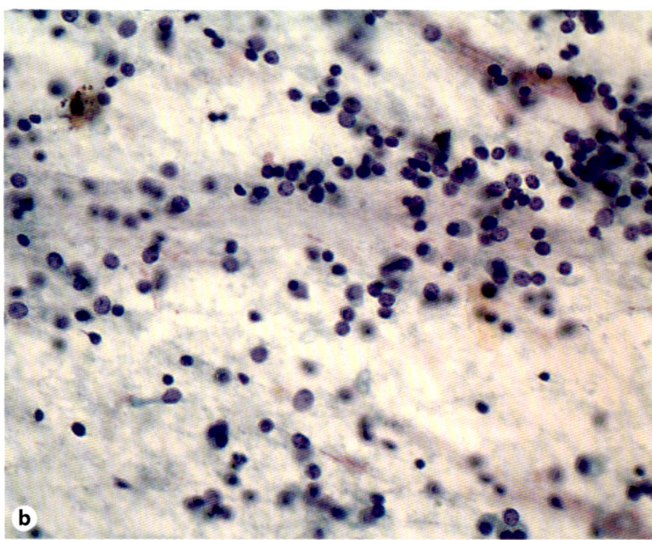

Fig. 3. Smear preparation artifacts including crush and air drying render this smear from a low-grade neuroendocrine carcinoma uninterpretable (**a**). A well-prepared area from another smear from the same tumor highlights distinctive diagnostic features of low-grade neuroendocrine carcinoma including plasmacytoid morphology and eccentric nuclei with characteristic neuroendocrine chromatin (**b**).

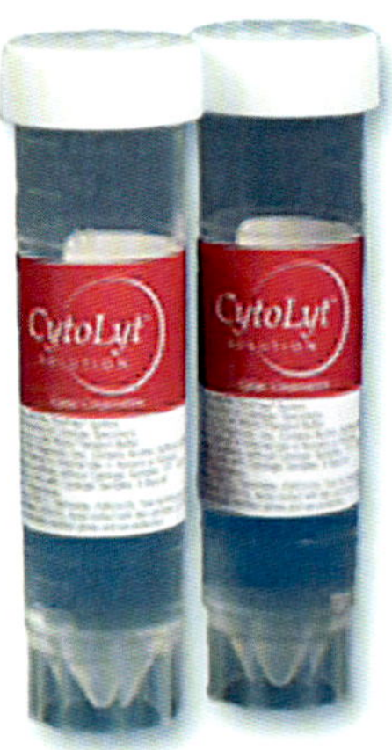

Fig. 4. Needle rinse samples are commonly obtained from ocular aspirates. These preparations have a concentration step prior to slide preparation. Material may be placed in Cytolyt solution for Thinprep processing. The same Thinprep slide can be used for diagnosis and for fluorescence in situ hybridization testing if indicated.

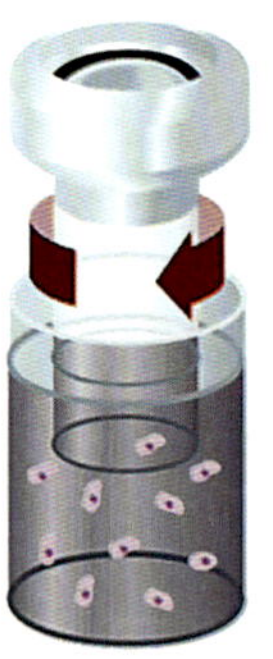

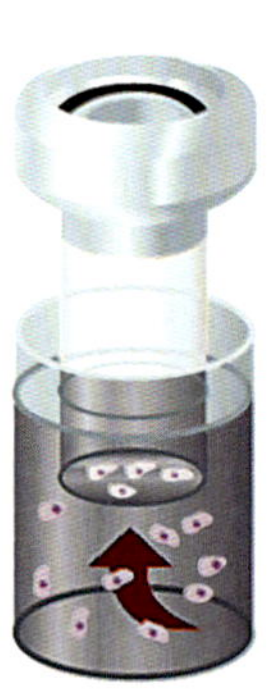

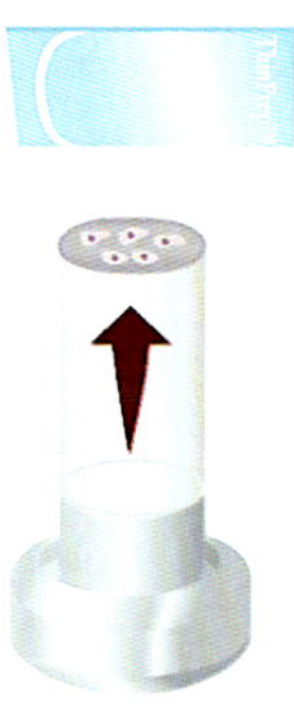

Fig. 5. Automated Thinprep processing. The Thinprep filter rotates in the sample separating cellular material from background debris. A vacuum collects cells on the exterior surface of the filter membrane. The filter is then inverted and gently pressed against the Thinprep slide. Surface tension and air pressure cause the cells to adhere to the slide, resulting in even distribution of cells in a central circular region of the slide.

is resuspended in a cell preservative solution, Preservcyt® for automated processing. The Thinprep processor mixes the sample and then, using a gentle vacuum, collects cells on a filter in an evenly dispersed way, approaching a monolayer. This filter is then inverted and its cellular contents transferred to a microscope slide (fig. 5). This method optimizes cell yield and preservation and standardizes slide preparation for interpretation in this setting of limited material. Also, if the sample is diagnostic of ocular melanoma or lymphoma, fluorescence in situ hybridization (FISH) testing for chromosomal abnormalities can be done on Thinprep slides (fig. 6). If abundant aspirate material is obtained or a sample is clotted or shows particles floating in the rinse solution, processing a paraffin-embedded cell block is also an option. Paraffin-embedded cell blocks are processed like surgical biopsy specimens and stained with a standard hematoxylin and eosin

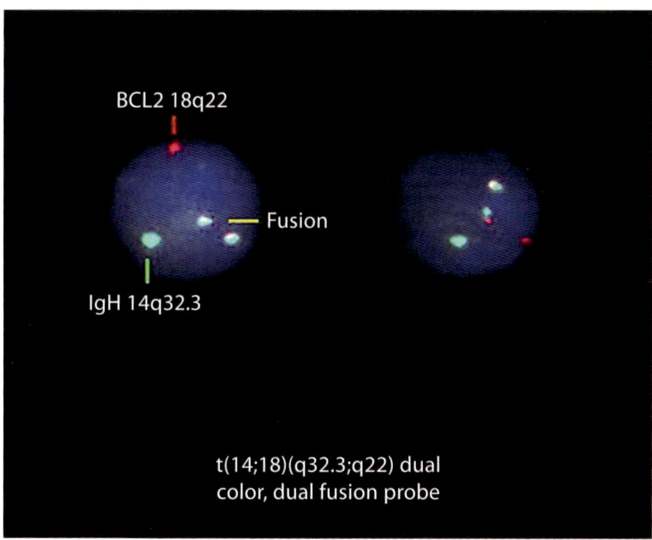

Fig. 6. FISH performed on a Thinprep slide shows a positive result for the translocation characteristic of follicular lymphoma t(14;18) (q32.3;q22). The same slide used for diagnosis can be submitted for FISH testing.

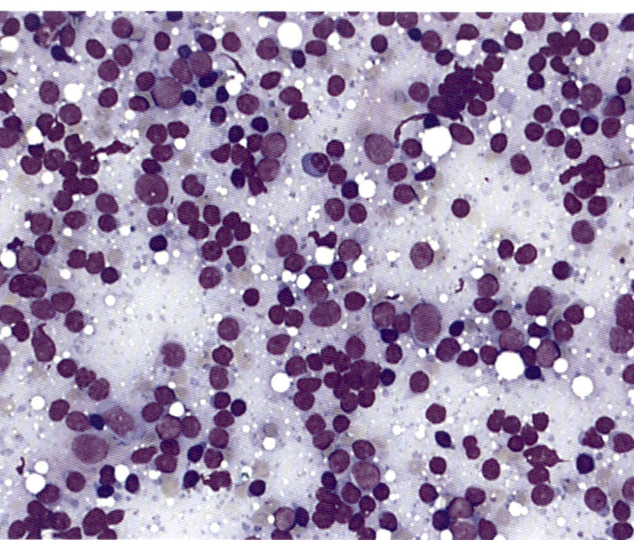

Fig. 8. An air-dried Diff-Quik stain from a reactive lymphoid sample highlights a mixed population of lymphocytes and plasma cells and background lymphoglandular bodies. The Diff-Quik stain is a rapid stain commonly used for on-site adequacy assessments.

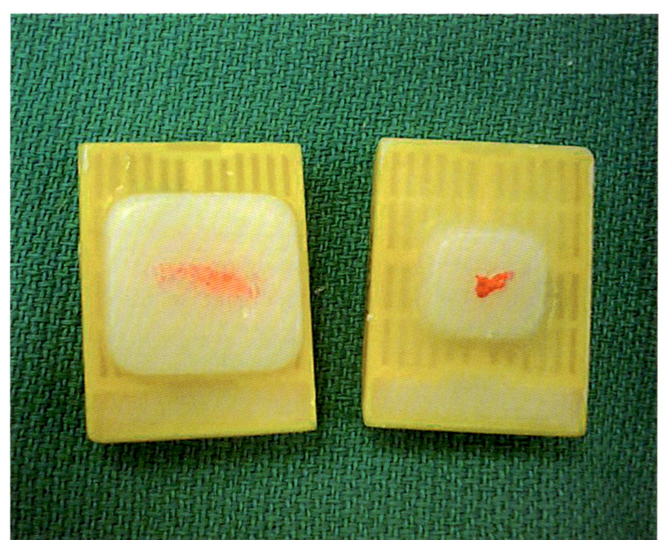

Fig. 7. Paraffin-embedded cell blocks are processed like surgical biopsy specimens and are cut and stained with hematoxylin and eosin. These cell blocks are the best source of material for immunohistochemistry.

stain. Paraffin-embedded cell block sections provide the best substrate for immunohistochemical staining (fig. 7). While at our institution we rarely perform immunostains on preparations other than a cell block, some authors have reported successful immunohistochemical analyses on thin-layer cytology preparations, cytospins and direct smears in limited samples [7–9].

Fixation and Staining

Aspirate samples may be air dried or immediately placed in 95% ethanol fixative. Immediate alcohol fixation while the smear is still wet is required to prevent air-drying artifacts from compromising the sample [3, 5]. Air-dried smears are stained with a Romanovsky method. Romanovsky stains include May-Grünwald-Giemsa, Wright and Diff-Quik stains. If a cytologist is on site during the aspiration procedure to render an opinion on specimen adequacy, a rapid Romanovsky stain such as the Diff-Quik, which takes less than 1 min, is generally used (fig. 8). Air-dried, Romanovsky-stained preparations have the advantage of highlighting background matrix/stromal material and cytoplasmic features [2]. Fixed slides are stained with the Papanicolaou (Pap) stain. The Pap stain highlights nuclear features and has the advantage of sharp chromatin detail. If the sample is limited, the Pap stain provides the best cellular detail for diagnosis (fig. 9) [5].

After smears have been prepared, most operators rinse the needle in a preservative solution to enhance cell yield.

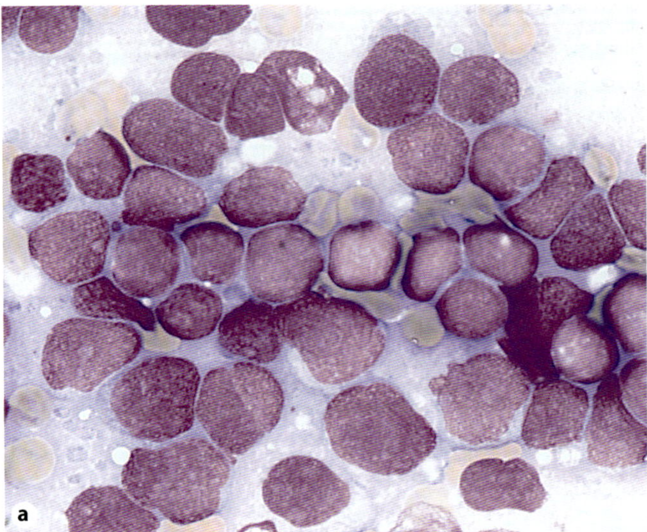

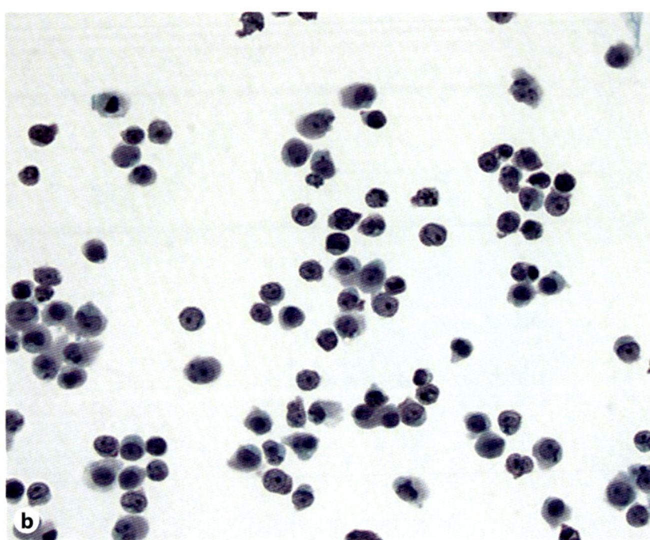

Fig. 9. Another Romanovsky stain, the Wright stain of a diffuse large B-cell lymphoma. Romanovsky type stains, including Wright and Diff-Quik, highlight background material, stroma and cytoplasmic features. These stains are quite helpful in hematolymphoid samples (**a**). The same large cell lymphoma stained with Pap stain. The Pap stain is performed on alcohol-fixed slides. Note the chromatin detail and prominent nucleoli (**b**).

In a patient with a known or suspected lymphoproliferative disorder, the needle may be rinsed into a cellular nutrient medium such as Roswell Park Medical Institution (RPMI) medium, for flow cytometry. In order to obtain sufficient numbers of lymphoid cells for flow cytometry, at least one dedicated pass should be entirely placed in RPMI medium (fig. 10). Flow cytometry cannot be reliably performed on alcohol-preserved aspirate samples.

Interpretation

After slides have been prepared, they are generally screened by a certified cytotechnologist and then reviewed by a cytopathologist for the final diagnosis. Either at this time or at the time of on-site adequacy assessment, decisions are made about additional necessary testing including immunohistochemistry and FISH. Cytopathologists interpreting ocular FNA are ideally in close communication with the operating ophthalmologist regarding history and clinical and radiological findings. The ideal cytopathologist is experienced and has knowledge of ocular histology and intraocular pathology [8, 10]. In some institutions, a cytopathologist is present on site during the FNA procedure to assess specimen adequacy. This rapid on-site evaluation has been shown to reduce the number of unsatisfactory aspirate samples [8, 9, 11, 12]. However, more than one aspirate sample may be needed to obtain a fully diagnostic sample in a subset of patients.

In addition to diagnostic confirmation, specimens from uveal melanoma obtained by FNA may provide useful prognostic information. Specifically, monosomy of chromosome 3 and chromosome 8q amplification have proven to be significantly associated with poor prognosis [13]. FISH is a reliable method for detecting these abnormalities in FNA samples. In our laboratory, the same Thinprep slides used for diagnosis are submitted for FISH analysis using centromeric probes for chromosome 3 and the 8q24 MYC locus [14]. In general, 2 Pap-stained Thinprep slides, ideally containing at least 200 tumor cells, are submitted for FISH analysis. This has proven to be an accurate method for testing that allows for maximum use of small samples [Chapter 6, this vol., pp. 55–60] [14].

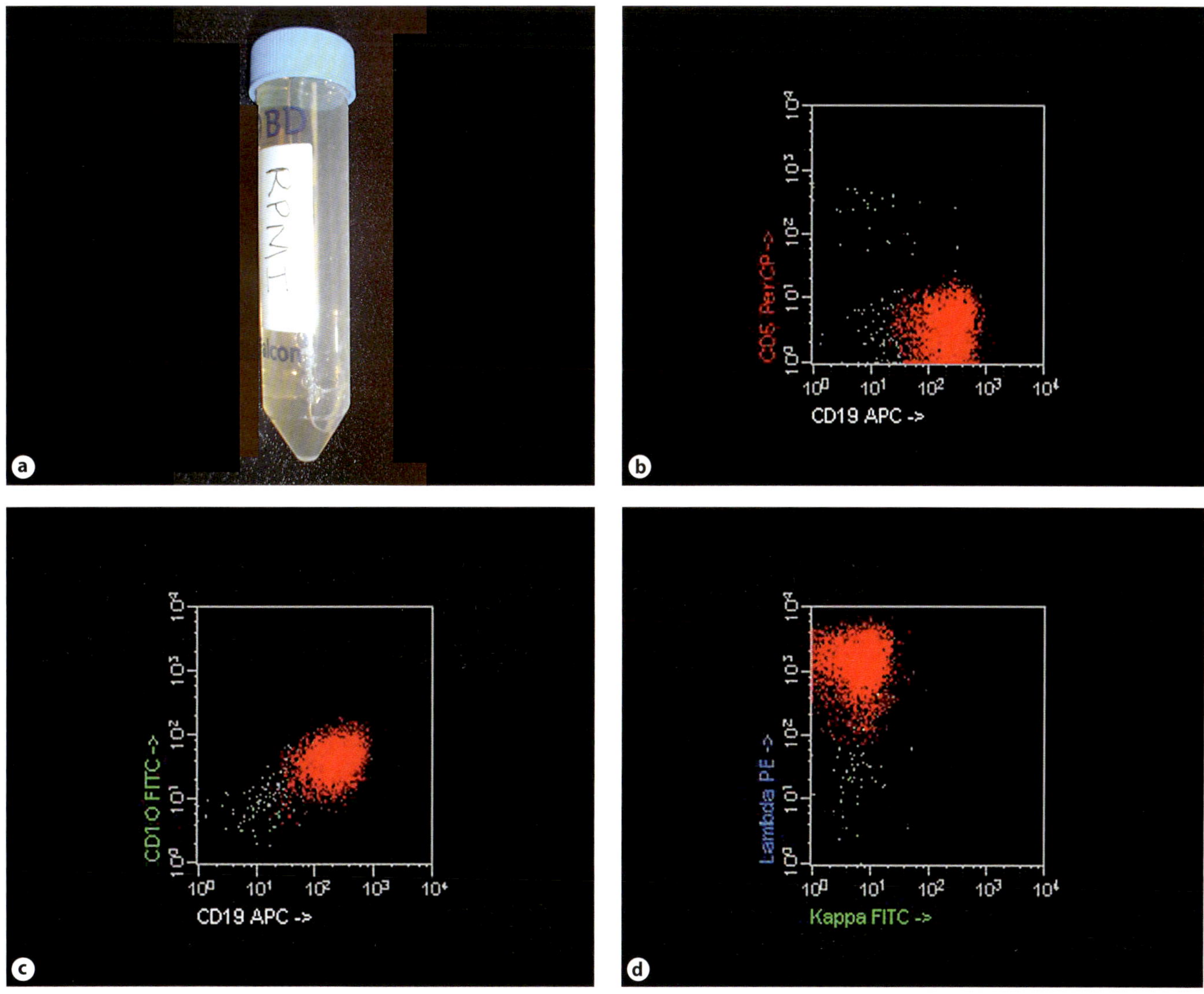

Fig. 10. If a lymphoproliferative disorder is suspected clinically or based on adequacy assessment, the needle should be rinsed in a cell preservative solution, such as RPMI medium to allow for flow cytometry (**a**). Flow cytometry performed on an FNA sample shows a monoclonal lymphoid population coexpressing CD10, CD19 and demonstrating λ light chain restriction in a patient with follicular lymphoma (**b–d**).

References

1 Frable WJ: Needle aspiration biopsy: past, present, and future. Hum Pathol 1989;20:504–517.
2 Ansari NA, Derias NW: Fine needle aspiration cytology. J Clin Pathol 1997;50:541–543.
3 Wu M, Burstein DE: Fine needle aspiration. Cancer Invest 2004;22:620–628.
4 Rosa M: Fine-needle aspiration biopsy: a historical overview. Diagn Cytopathol 2008;36:773–775.
5 Frable WJ: Fine-needle aspiration biopsy: a review. Hum Pathol 1983;14:9–28.
6 Hoda RS: Non-gynecologic cytology on liquid-based preparations: a morphologic review of facts and artifacts. Diagn Cytopathol 2007;35:621–634.
7 Pelayes DE, Zarate JO: Fine needle aspiration biopsy with liquid-based cytology and adjunct immunohistochemistry in intraocular melanocytic tumors. Eur J Ophthalmol 2010;20:1059–1065.
8 Faulkner-Jones BE, Foster WJ, Harbour JW, Smith ME, Davila RM: Fine needle aspiration biopsy with adjunct immunohistochemistry in intraocular tumor management. Acta Cytol 2005;49:297–308.
9 Eide N, Walaas L: Fine-needle aspiration biopsy and other biopsies in suspected intraocular malignant disease: a review. Acta Ophthalmol 2009;87:588–601.

10 Shields JA, Shields CL, Ehya H, Eagle RC Jr, De Potter P: Fine-needle aspiration biopsy of suspected intraocular tumors: the 1992 Urwick lecture. Ophthalmology 1993;100:1677–1684.
11 Char DH, Kemlitz AE, Miller T: Intraocular biopsy. Ophthalmol Clin North Am 2005;18:177–185.
12 Augsburger JJ: Fine needle aspiration biopsy of suspected metastatic cancers to the posterior uvea. Trans Am Ophthalmol Soc 1988;86:499–560.
13 Singh AD, Tubbs R, Biscotti C, Schoenfield L, Trizzoi P: Chromosomal 3 and 8 status within hepatic metastasis of uveal melanoma. Arch Pathol Lab Med 2009;133:1223–1227.
14 Skacel M, Pettay JD, Tsiftsakis EK, Procop GW, Biscotti CV, Tubbs RR: Validation of a multicolor interphase fluorescence in situ hybridization assay for detection of transitional cell carcinoma on fresh and archival thin-layer, liquid-based cytology slides. Anal Quant Cytol Histol 2001;23: 381–387.

Charles V. Biscotti, MD
Department of Anatomic Pathology, Cleveland Clinic Foundation
9500 Euclid Avenue
Cleveland, OH 44195 (USA)
Tel. +1 216 444 0046, E-Mail biscotc@ccf.org

Chapter 3
Biscotti CV, Singh AD (eds): FNA Cytology of Ophthalmic Tumors.
Monogr Clin Cytol. Basel, Karger 2012, vol 21, pp 17–30

Uveal Metastases

Charles V. Biscotti[a] · Arun D. Singh[b]
Departments of [a]Anatomic Pathology and [b]Ophthalmology, Cleveland Clinic Foundation, Cleveland, Ohio, USA

Any discussion of ophthalmic oncology must emphasize metastases to the uvea. Consider that an estimated 8–10% of patients with metastatic malignancy have uveal involvement [1]. Not surprisingly then, metastases are the most common uveal malignancy. The uveal tract's rich vascularity partly explains this predilection for metastases. Further, the uveal microenvironment seems favorable to metastases since the uvea has the highest percentage of metastatic involvement in relation to blood flow of any tissue in the body [1, 2]. Metastases usually involve the choroid (88% of cases) and rarely involve the iris (9% of cases) or ciliary body (2% of cases) [3]. Multifocality and or bilaterality can help clinically differentiate metastases from primary tumors, especially melanoma. Unfortunately, metastases are often solitary and unilateral [3, 4]. In one large series, metastases were bilateral in only approximately one quarter of patients, and the metastases were solitary in 71% of the involved eyes [3]. Two thirds of patients with uveal metastases have a history of a primary malignancy [3]. Cytologists should exploit this fact when interpreting uveal fine needle aspiration biopsy (FNAB) samples.

Clinical Features

Breast and lung carcinoma dominate the primary malignancies that metastasize to the uvea. The breast is the most common primary site in women and the lung is the most common primary site in men [3–6]. In a large series of uveal metastases, the distribution of primary sites included the breast (47% of cases), lung (21% of cases) and gastrointestinal tract (4% of cases) [3]. Interestingly, the lung is the most likely primary site of uveal metastatic carcinoma in patients with no known primary at presentation [3, 7–10]. In one large series, one third of patients had no history of primary malignancy at the time of diagnosis of their uveal metastasis. Subsequent evaluation identified a lung primary (35% of patients), breast primary (7% of patients) and other primary sites (6% of patients) [3]. In this series, a primary site was not detected in 17% of patients overall [3], which is higher than the 5% reported rate of unknown primaries in the general oncological literature [11].

Symptomatic choroidal metastases precede the diagnosis of the lung primary in most (64%) patients [7]. In contrast, uveal metastases from breast carcinoma usually occur late in the natural history and are associated with disseminated disease in patients with a known breast primary [4, 12]. Importantly, sarcomas rarely metastasize to the uvea [5], a fact that should be considered when facing a malignant spindle cell neoplasm in a uveal FNAB sample. In this instance, spindle cell melanoma should be considered in the diagnosis.

Peculiarities of uveal metastases from renal cell carcinoma can cause diagnostic problems. Firstly, uveal metastasis may precede the diagnosis of a renal primary in approximately 48% of cases [13]. Further, renal cell carcinoma can metastasize after long latency periods. Uveal metastasis has been reported more than 16 years after the primary diagnosis of renal cell carcinoma [13]. Cytologists should consider renal cell carcinoma given a uveal lesion, clinically suspicious for metastasis, that does not resemble the usual breast or lung carcinoma, especially in the presence of cellular features characteristic of clear cell differentiation, that is abundant finely vacuolated cytoplasm and relatively bland nuclei often

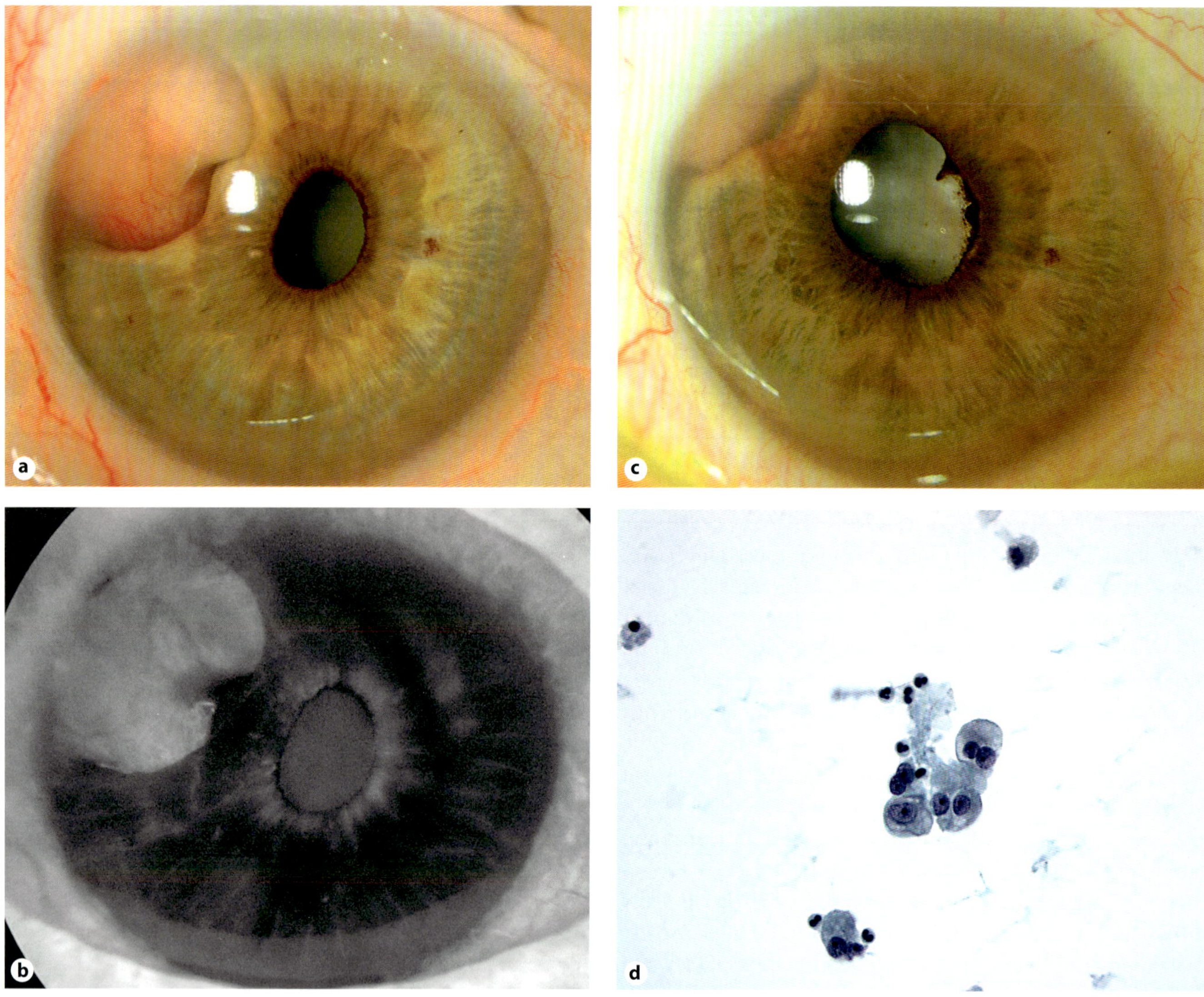

Fig. 1. A 68-year-old man initially presented with left hip pain which led to a diagnosis of left renal mass with widespread bone metastasis. Left radical nephrectomy showed evidence of clear cell type renal cell carcinoma (grade 4). There was evidence of penetration of the renal capsule and infiltration of perinephric fat and invasion of the renal vein. He was treated with interferon α, local radiation therapy and Zometa. He continued to progress slowly despite being treated with several investigational drugs developing ocular pain 4 years later. On examination visual acuity was 20/200 OD with normal intraocular pressure. A kidney-shaped vascular mass was visible in the iridociliary region (**a**). Anterior segment fluorescein angiography confirmed vascularity of the lesion (**b**). Four weeks following treatment with iodine-125 plaque radiotherapy, marked regression of the lesion is evident (**c**). FNAB of metastatic renal cell carcinoma illustrates the characteristic features of clear cell renal cell carcinoma (**d**). Note the abundant finely vacuolated cytoplasm surrounding nuclei with prominent nucleoli.

containing conspicuous nucleoli (fig. 1). Metastatic renal cell carcinoma can be overlooked because of these typical cellular features, especially the bland nuclei and low nuclear-to-cytoplasmic ratio. In particular, renal cell carcinoma can be misinterpreted as a xanthogranulomatous inflammatory reaction. Cognizance of the clinical and cellular features can help avoid this pitfall.

Diagnostic Evaluation

Diagnostic FNAB is indicated in only an estimated 2.5% of patients with intraocular tumors overall and up to 7% of patients with iris tumors [14, 15]. However, FNAB has a well-established role in the diagnosis of uveal metastases, especially when a primary malignancy is not known

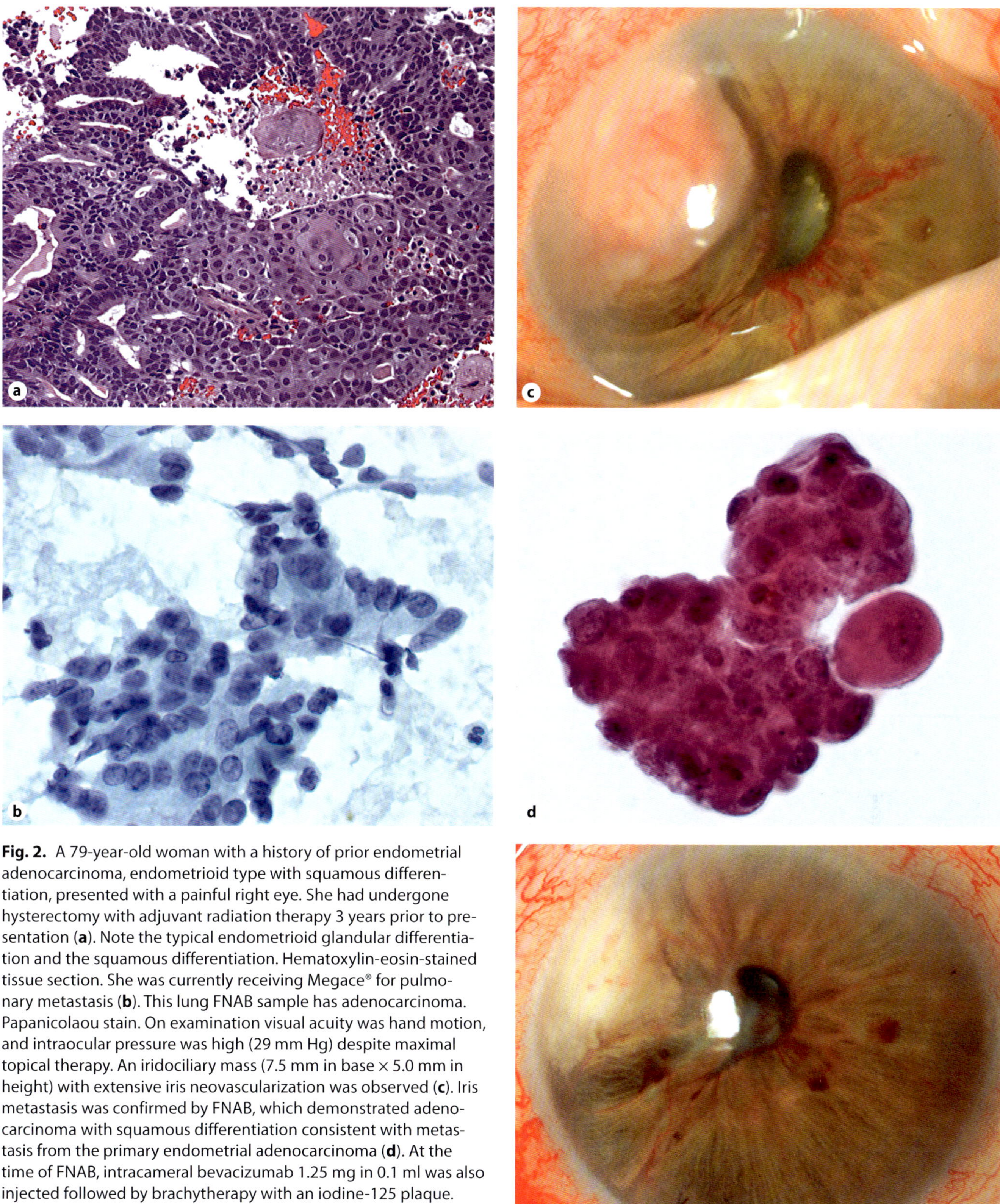

Fig. 2. A 79-year-old woman with a history of prior endometrial adenocarcinoma, endometrioid type with squamous differentiation, presented with a painful right eye. She had undergone hysterectomy with adjuvant radiation therapy 3 years prior to presentation (**a**). Note the typical endometrioid glandular differentiation and the squamous differentiation. Hematoxylin-eosin-stained tissue section. She was currently receiving Megace® for pulmonary metastasis (**b**). This lung FNAB sample has adenocarcinoma. Papanicolaou stain. On examination visual acuity was hand motion, and intraocular pressure was high (29 mm Hg) despite maximal topical therapy. An iridociliary mass (7.5 mm in base × 5.0 mm in height) with extensive iris neovascularization was observed (**c**). Iris metastasis was confirmed by FNAB, which demonstrated adenocarcinoma with squamous differentiation consistent with metastasis from the primary endometrial adenocarcinoma (**d**). At the time of FNAB, intracameral bevacizumab 1.25 mg in 0.1 ml was also injected followed by brachytherapy with an iodine-125 plaque. Four weeks after the treatment, the ocular pain had subsided with dramatic shrinkage of the tumor (**e**). In addition there was complete regression of iris neovascularization with normalization of intraocular pressure.

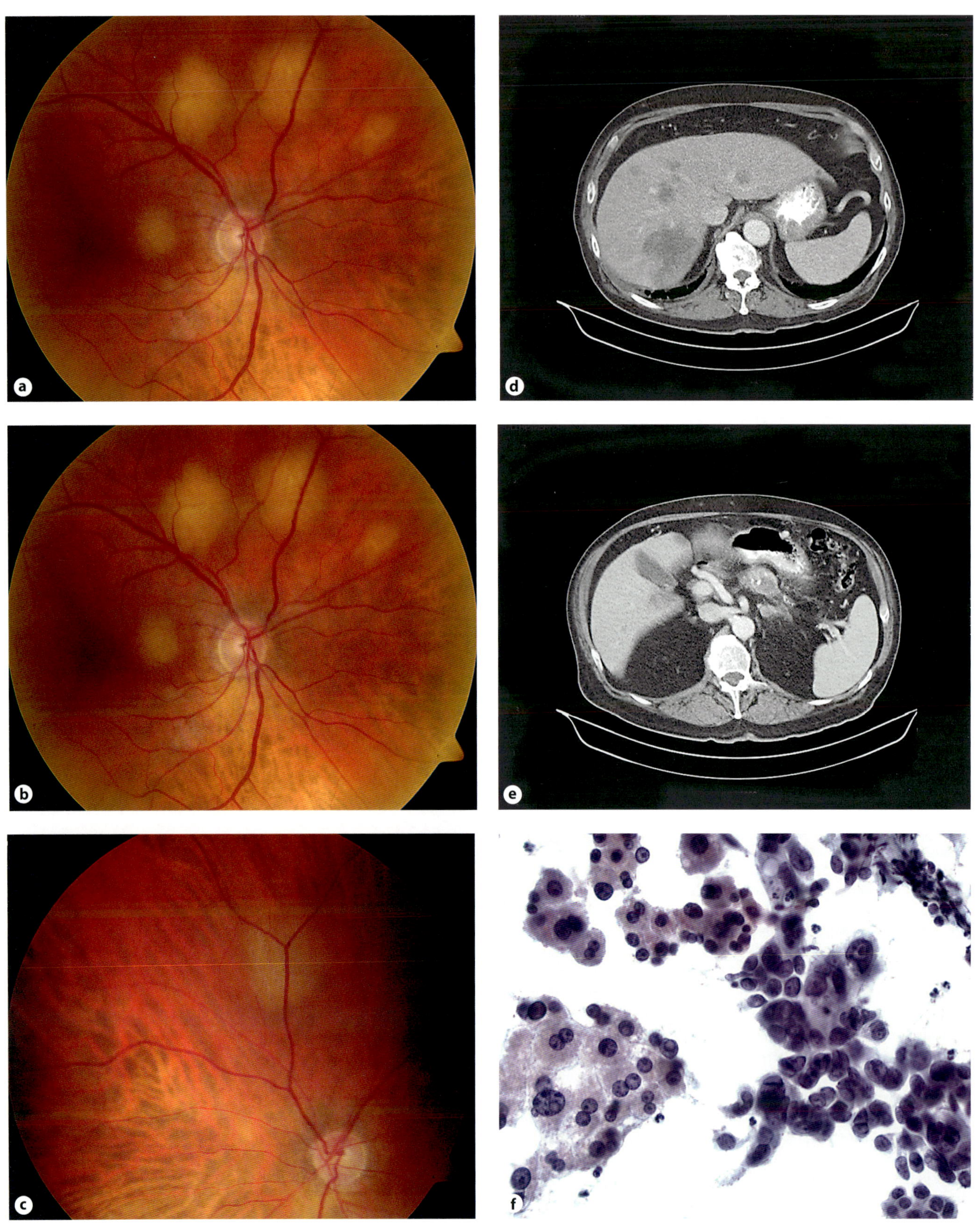
a
b
c
d
e
f

(approx. one third of patients) or in those rare cases with contentious clinical findings [5, 16, 17].

The most common indications for uveal FNAB are confirmation of a clinical suspicion of metastasis and resolution of the rare ambiguous case of metastasis versus melanoma [5]. In three series, 86–90% of diagnostic FNAB samples were judged adequate [5, 16, 18]. The positive predictive value of FNAB, especially given a clinical impression of malignancy, is excellent, and a positive diagnosis is reliable for clinical management. We agree with others that a negative result should be interpreted with caution and not considered proof of a benign process [19, 20]. In our experience and that of others, given a clinical impression of metastasis or metastasis versus melanoma, an insufficient or negative FNAB result should trigger a repeat FNAB [16].

Differential Diagnosis

The indications for uveal FNAB should frame any discussion of the cytological differential diagnosis of uveal masses [6, 19]. Cytologists should always look for a history of primary malignancy when analyzing uveal FNAB specimens. If available, any prior cytological or histological material should be reviewed for comparison. In our experience, this comparison almost always confirms the diagnosis and obviates the need for other corroborative tests such as immunohistochemistry (fig. 2–4). The value of morphological comparison is especially true for metastatic breast carcinoma which typically resembles the primary tumor in any of its metastatic sites (fig. 5).

Remember that when the primary site is unknown, lung carcinoma is the most likely primary (fig. 6). Residual cells in the needle rinse tend to be limited in uveal aspirate samples restricting immunohistochemistry options. So, cytologists should prioritize corroborative immunohistochemistry with these facts in mind. Specifically, when the cellular features are suggestive, employing thyroid transcription factor 1, which should be positive in lung adenocarcinoma and small cell carcinoma (fig. 7).

Similarly, cellular features are usually sufficient to resolve the metastasis versus melanoma differential diagnosis. Since metastases are almost always carcinoma, they show cellular features of epithelial differentiation, notably cellular cohesion (fig. 7). In contrast, melanomas have an individual cell pattern (fig. 8) [Chapter 5, this vol., pp. 44–54]. Further, melanomas have a characteristic constellation of cellular features including at least a component of spindle cells and relatively bland nuclei compared to metastases (fig. 9) [18, 24]. Rarely, high nuclear grade epithelioid melanomas can mimic metastatic carcinoma. Cytokeratin and S100 immunostains are useful in this instance. Prostate-specific antigen immunostain can help corroborate the diagnosis of metastatic prostate carcinoma (fig. 10).

Other differential diagnostic considerations include lymphoma, leukemia and leiomyoma [Chapter 4, this vol., pp. 31–43]. Cellular samples containing lymphoma or leukemia lack the cell-to-cell articulation characteristic of metastatic carcinoma. Immunohistochemical stains for cytokeratins and a broad spectrum lymphoid marker such as common leukocyte antigen can help in problematic cases. Finally, cellular samples from leiomyomas have a dispersed spindle cell pattern which contrasts with the pattern characteristic of metastatic carcinoma.

Fig. 3. A 71-year-old man who presented with blurred vision in the right eye for the last 2 months. Personal history, family history and social history were noncontributory. On examination, the visual acuity was 20/50 in both eyes. Fundus evaluation of the right eye showed multiple scattered subretinal pale lesions (**a**). The largest one was in the temporal macula and measured about 7 × 6 × 2 mm (**b**). The left eye also showed 2 small lesions (**c**). The clinical findings suggested metastases. CT scan of the chest, abdomen and pelvis revealed numerous lesions throughout the right and left hepatic lobes (**d**). A soft tissue mass with calcification was identified in the region of the pancreatic body measuring 5 × 3.2 cm (**e**). Hepatic FNAB confirmed adenocarcinoma consistent with metastatic pancreatic ductal carcinoma (**f**). Note that the hepatocytes, to the left, have abundant granular cytoplasm. These sharply contrast with the adenocarcinoma cells, to the right, which have higher nuclear-to-cytoplasmic ratios and a crowded disorganized pattern. Papanicolaou stain.

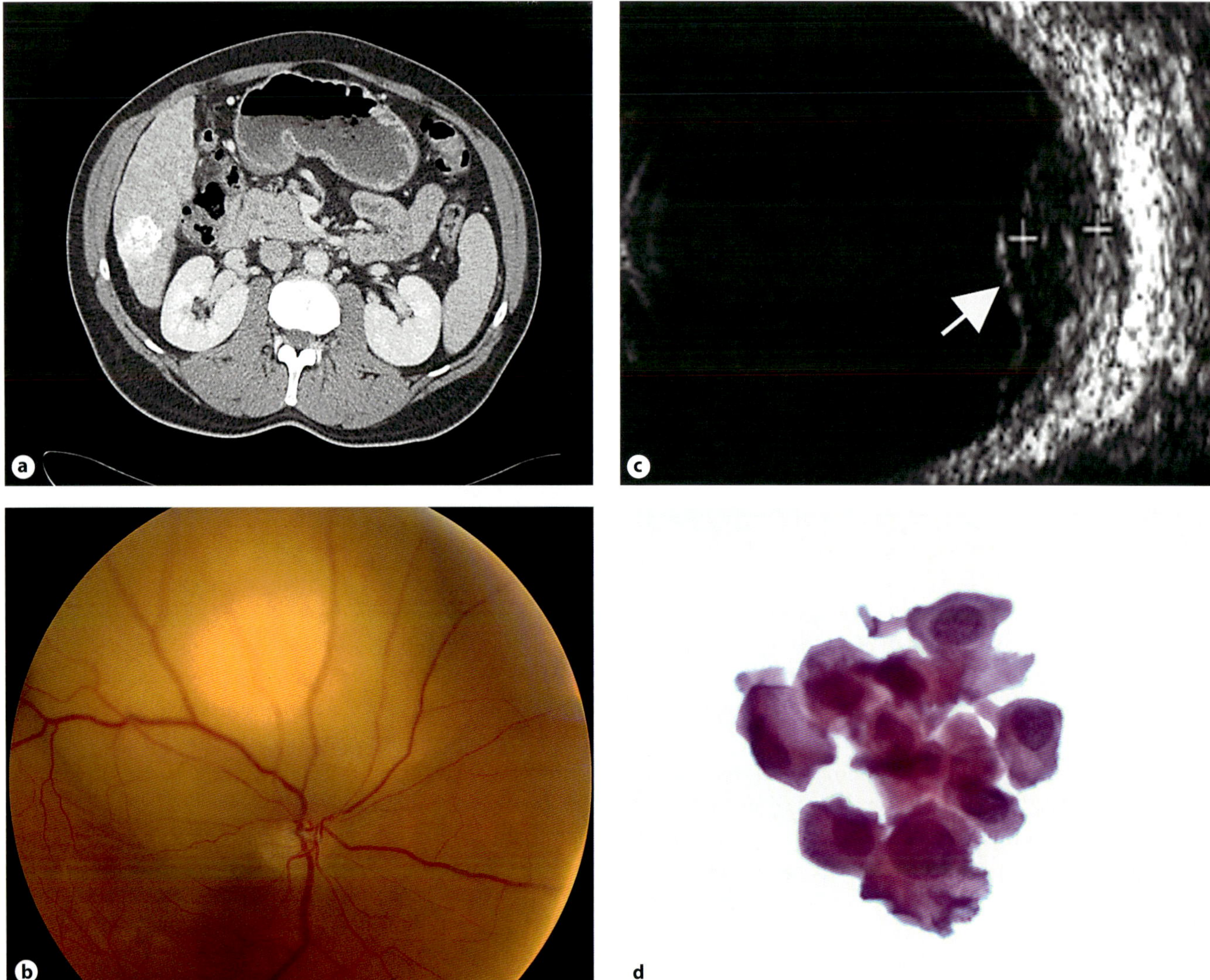

Fig. 4. A 57-year-old man, a chronic alcohol abuser, with a 3-year history of untreated hepatitis C infection was found to have an elevated α-fetoprotein concentration of 62.3 ng/ml on routine follow-up. Abdominal MRI was consistent with the presence of liver cirrhosis and 2 suspicious masses in the posterior inferior right lobe of the liver (**a**). The patient subsequently underwent a biopsy of the larger of the 2 lesions, which was positive for moderately differentiated hepatocellular carcinoma and was treated with 1 course of Therasphere® administration to the left liver lobe. About 5 months later, the patient complained of a 2-week history of progressive blurry vision OD. Ophthalmoscopic examination showed a yellow-white dome-shaped choroidal mass abutting the optic disk with surrounding shallow exudative retinal detachment (**b**). Ocular B-scan ultrasonography confirmed a dome-shaped choroidal mass (between calipers) with overlying retinal detachment (arrow; **c**). Extrascleral extension was absent. The patient then underwent FNAB of the mass, which revealed the presence of carcinoma cells consistent with metastatic hepatocellular carcinoma (**d**; Thinprep, Hologic Corp.). Hematoxylin and eosin. ×40. Restaging CT scanning of the chest, abdomen and pelvis showed no other possible primary site of tumor. The patient was treated with brachytherapy (iodine-125 radioactive episcleral plaque, 16 mm size, apical dose 43.33 Gy in 74 h). The patient died 3 weeks following therapy due to pneumonia. Reproduced with permission from Wesolowski et al. [21].

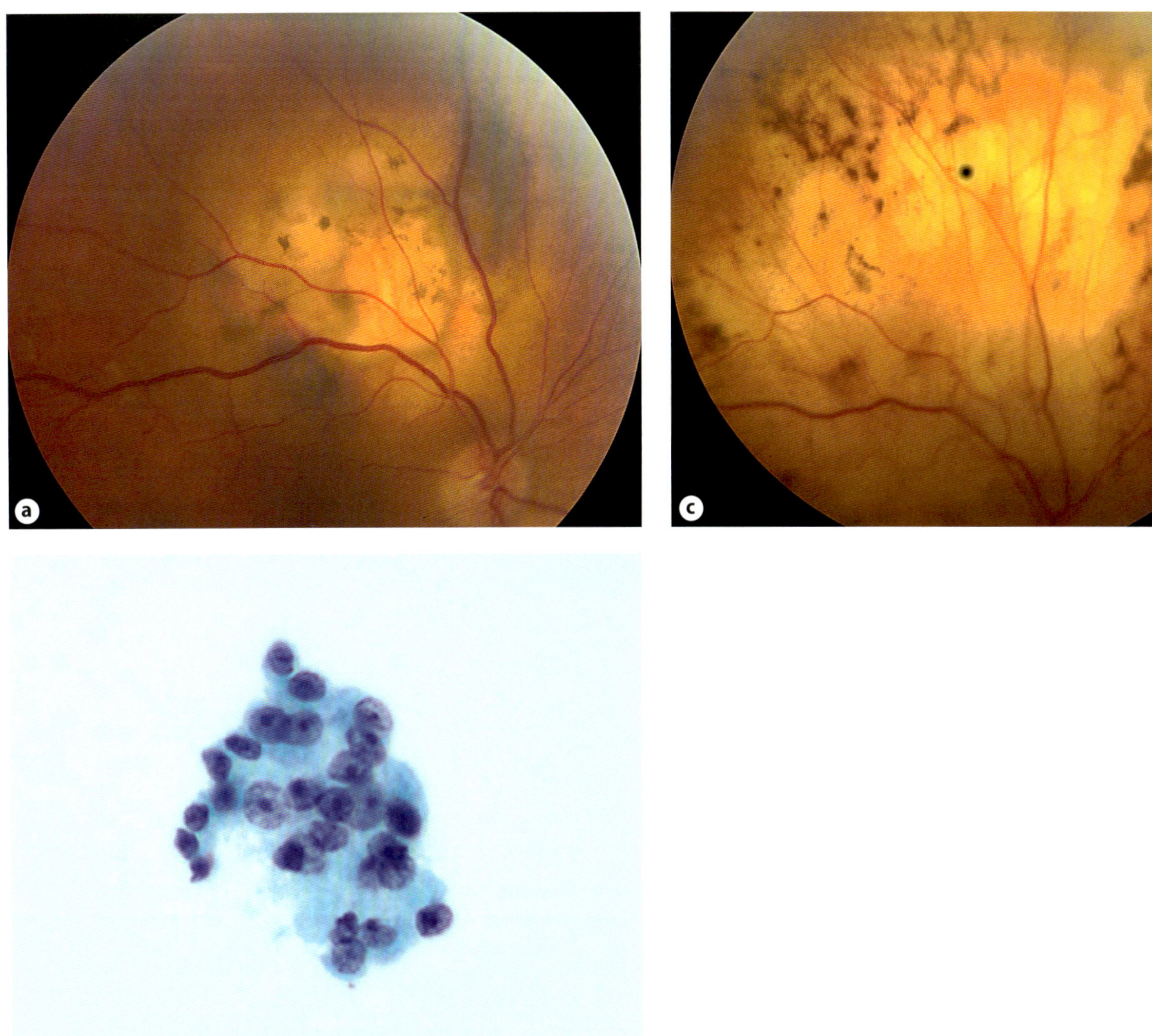

Fig. 5. A 76-year-old man underwent left modified radical mastectomy for adenocarcinoma of the left breast at an outside hospital; he did not receive any adjunctive treatment at the time of diagnosis. Approximately 2 years later, he was found to have a right axillary mass, which excisional biopsy demonstrated to be metastatic adenocarcinoma that was estrogen and progesterone receptor positive. Unfortunately, the patient was lost to follow-up. Two years later, the patient was referred for evaluation of blurred vision of several months' duration. Dilated fundus examination of the right eye revealed a single elevated creamy-white choroidal lesion in the superotemporal region (**a**). The left eye was normal. Standardized B-scan ultrasonography of the right eye demonstrated a placoid-shaped choroidal mass. An FNAB of the choroidal lesion confirmed adenocarcinoma consistent with metastasis from the breast (**b**, Papanicolaou stain). Restaging studies demonstrated new mediastinal and right hilar adenopathy, and a 1.8-cm peritoneal nodule. Bone scan also revealed 2 new focal lesions. In consultation with hematology-oncology, the patient was started on monthly intramuscular injections of goserelin 3.6 mg. After 5 months of treatment, letrozole 2.5 mg p.o. daily was added for progression of his pulmonary lesions. The choroidal metastasis showed initial regression for approximately 9 months before demonstrating marginal recurrence, at which point the patient underwent episcleral plaque brachytherapy application (iodine-125, 18 mm notched, 4,831 cGy, 71.5 h) to the right eye. For 5 months, the patient's choroidal metastasis remained clinically stable (**c**). However, the patient developed complications from progressive systemic metastases and died 1.5 years after his initial diagnosis of choroidal metastasis. Reproduced with permission from Hood et al. [22].

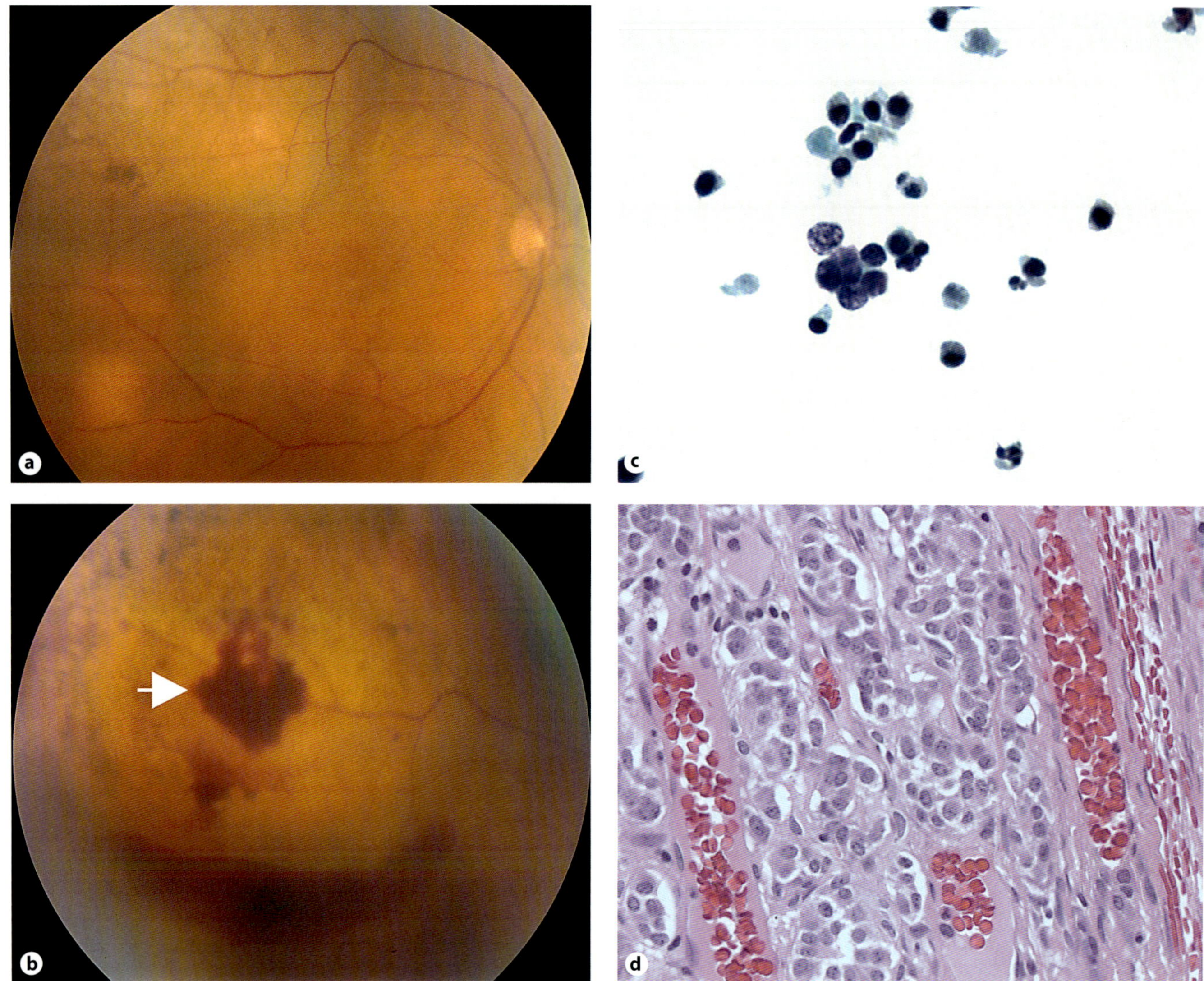

Fig. 6. A 79-year-old woman presented in May 2005 after reporting worsening vision OD. Visual acuity was 20/400 OD. Fundus examination at this time revealed 2 choroidal masses (**a**). The larger lesion, located off the superotemporal arcade, was 13 × 12 mm in basal diameter, 4.5 mm in height, and had loculated subretinal fluid with retinal pigment epithelium changes at the margins. She had been treated for disseminated small cell lung carcinoma since 2002. Standard chemotherapy consisting of carboplatin and etoposide was initiated with no radiological response. The patient subsequently had several lines of salvage chemotherapy including topotecan and paclitaxel with no radiological response. The absence of tumor progression cast doubt on the original diagnosis of small cell carcinoma, suggesting instead a carcinoid tumor. It was elected to proceed with transvitreal FNAB using a 25-gauge needle (**b**). Note the minimal vitreous and subretinal hemorrhage. The biopsy site (arrow) is plugged with a retinal hemorrhage. The FNAB yielded a cellular and relatively monomorphic sample consisting of mostly individual cells. The cells had bland nuclei with granular chromatin, often eccentrically placed in a moderate amount of cytoplasm. Note the individual cell pattern, eccentric nuclei and granular chromatin (**c**, Papanicolaou stain). The cellular features were characteristic of a low grade neuroendocrine carcinoma such as a carcinoid tumor. Cellular features of small cell carcinoma were not identified. The prior ovarian specimens also contained carcinoid tumor (**d**). The ovarian tissue specimens well illustrate the histological features of a low grade neuroendocrine carcinoma consistent with a metastatic carcinoid tumor. The cells are arranged in nests and cords. A moderate amount of eosinophilic cytoplasm surrounds relatively uniform nuclei with granular chromatin. Many of the tumor cells have eccentric nuclei and a plasmacytoid appearance. Note the absence of necrosis and mitoses. The patient underwent plaque radiotherapy using ruthenium-106. The patient also began treatment with octreotide in August 2005 and with partial resolution of chronic abdominal pain and nausea. At the last follow-up, the patient's visual acuity had improved to 20/200, and fundus examination showed resolution of subretinal fluid and reduction in lesion height to 3.4 mm. The patient died in February 2006, after a progressive decline in health. Reproduced with permission from Pelayes et al. [23].

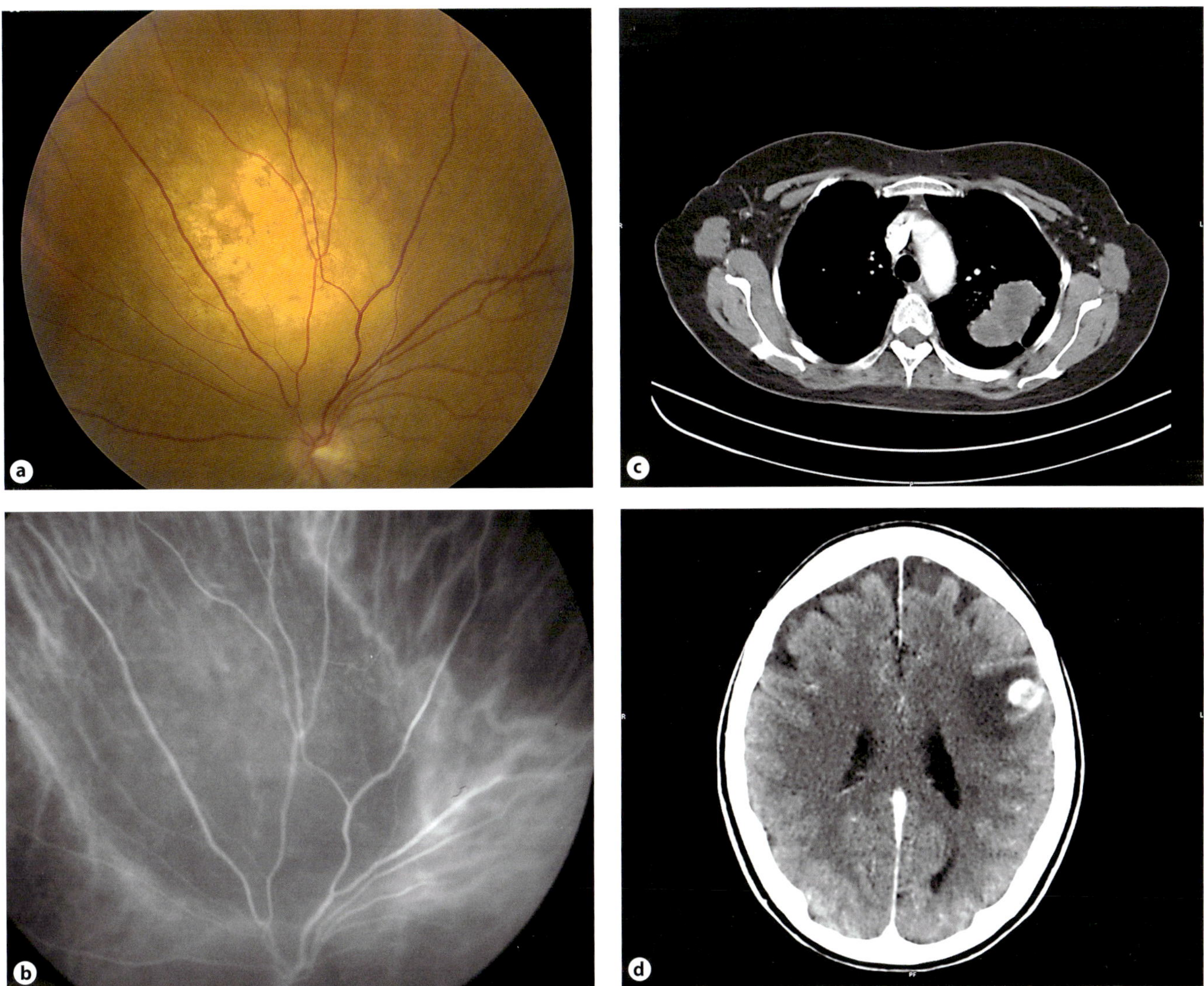

Fig. 7. A 56-year-old woman presented with flashing light sensation in the left eye. Her medical history was noncontributory. She was not a smoker and was apparently in good health. Ophthalmic examination revealed visual acuity of 20/25 OU. A single yellow-colored choroidal mass was observed on fundus examination of the left eye (**a**). The mass was 10 × 9 mm in basal dimension with thickness of 2.5 mm. Indocyanine angiography showed absence of intrinsic choroidal vasculature (**b**). A possibility of choroidal metastasis was suspected, and CT scan of the chest, abdomen and pelvis was ordered. Left apical lung lesion suspicious for lung carcinoma was detected (**c**) in addition to a brain metastasis (**d**). The consulting radiologist determined that the lung lesion was not easily accessible by FNAB.

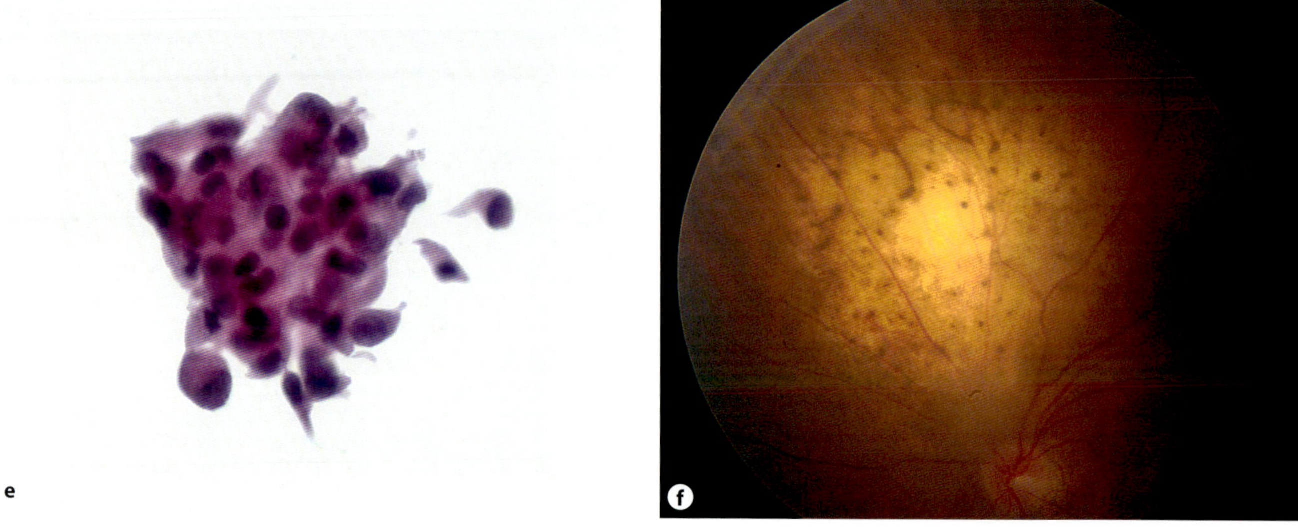

Fig. 7. Therefore, it was elected to proceed with FNAB of the choroidal lesion, which revealed adenocarcinoma (**e**). She was initially treated with whole brain radiation and Tarceva® that caused regression of the choroidal lesion (**f**), eventually requiring carboplatin and Taxol® for progressive metastatic disease.

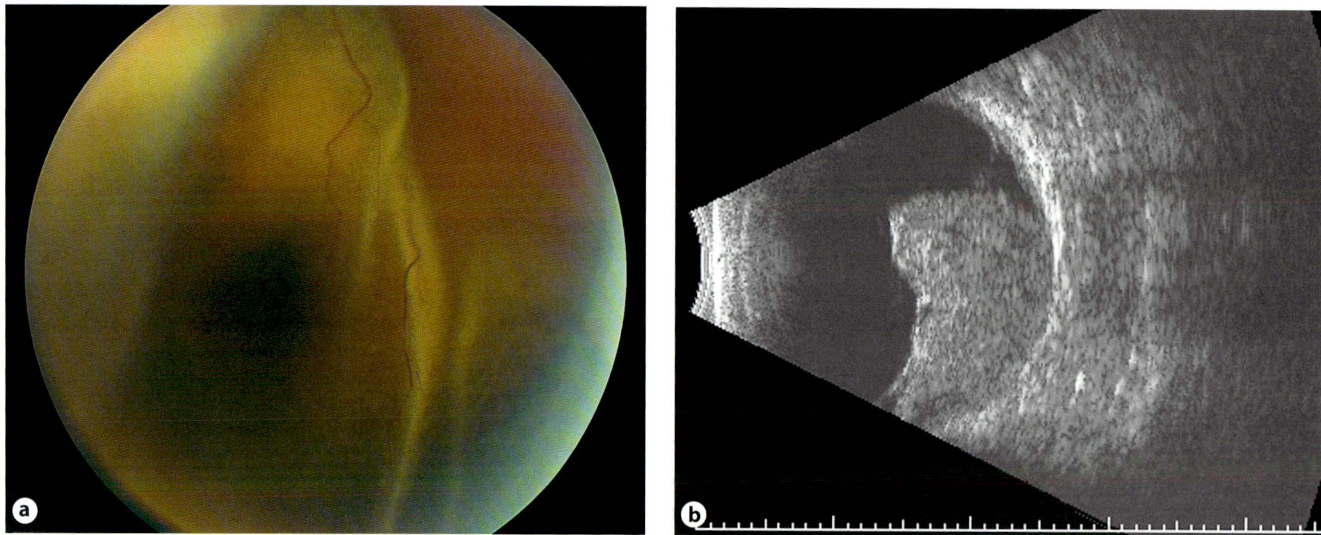

Fig. 8. A 69-year-old man was evaluated for floaters and flashing lights in the left eye for about 3 weeks' duration. He had a history of ischemic optic neuropathy with poor vision in the right eye (20/400) rendering him essentially monocular with vision of 20/30 in the left eye. On examination, a large pigmented multilobulated choroidal mass with exudative retinal detachment involving the nasal half of the fundus and overhanging the optic disk was observed (**a**). The size of the tumor was 24 × 18 in basal dimension with thickness of about 12 mm (**b**).

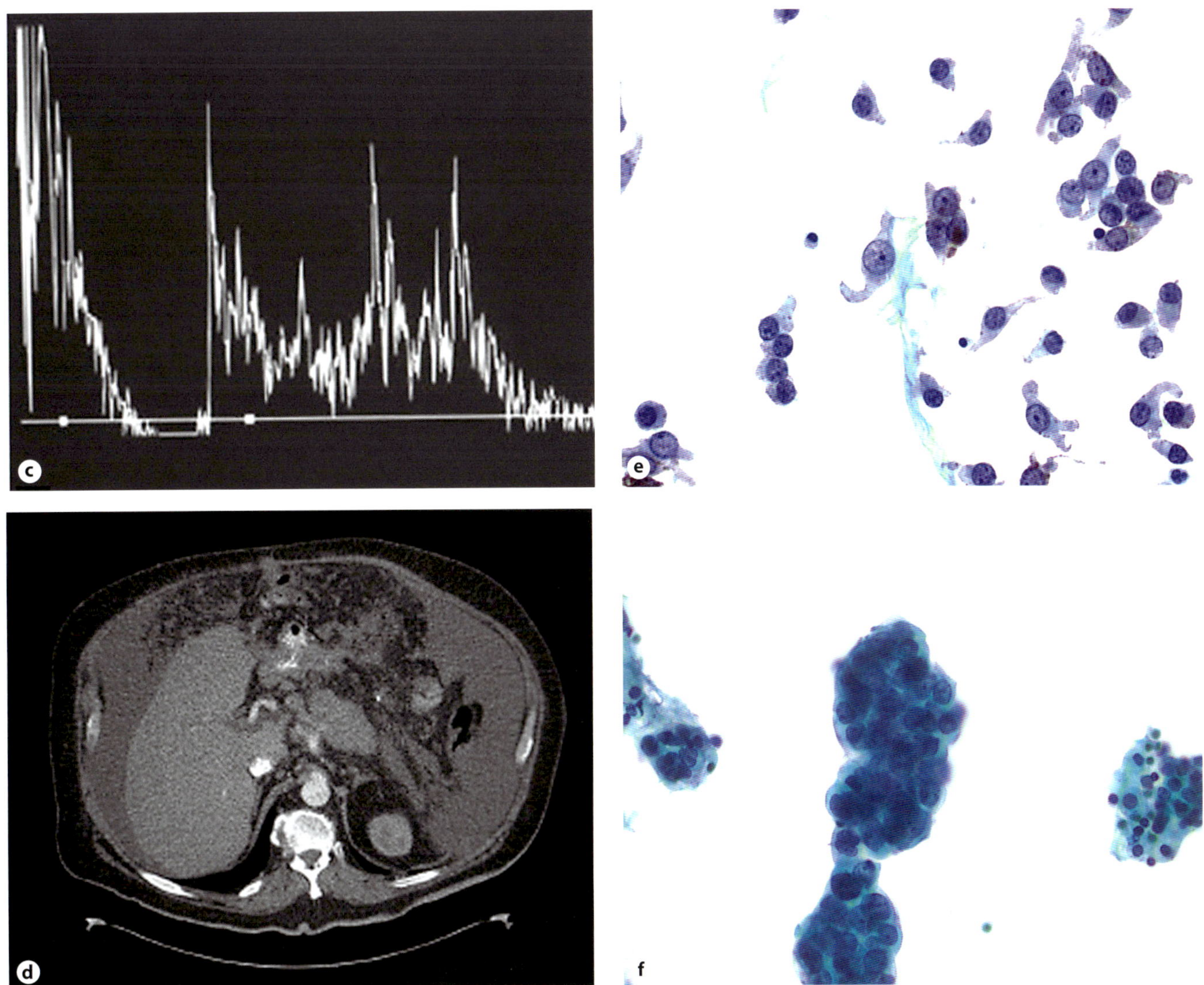

Fig. 8. Ultrasonography confirmed low to medium internal reflectivity suggestive of choroidal melanoma (**c**). Imaging studies to exclude metastasis revealed pancreatic mass raising doubts about the clinical diagnosis of the choroidal tumor (**d**). Diagnostic FNAB of the choroidal tumor confirmed the initial clinical suspicion of the choroidal melanoma (**e**). Note the individual cell pattern with spindle-shaped cells. The cells have nuclei with conspicuous nucleoli. Cytoplasmic pigment is evident though not prominent. Papanicolaou stain. Diagnostic paracentesis confirmed the presence of malignant ascites secondary to adenocarcinoma consistent with a pancreatic ductal primary (**f**, Papanicolaou stain). Given the overall poor prognosis for survival, choroidal melanoma was not treated. The patient died 9 weeks later.

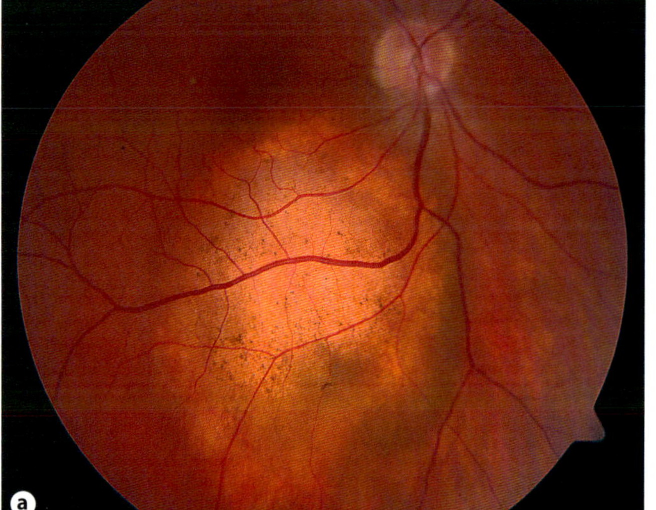

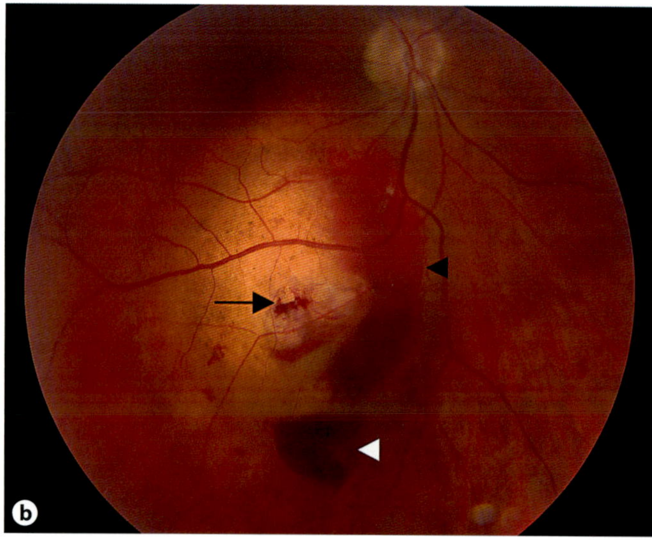

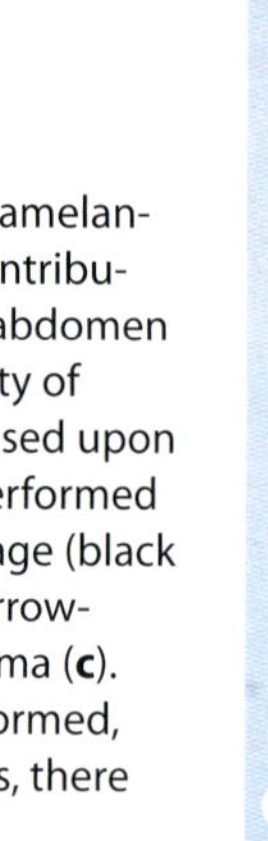

Fig. 9. A 42-year-old woman was evaluated for a partially amelanotic choroidal mass OD (**a**). Her medical history was noncontributory. Systemic evaluation including CT scans of the chest, abdomen and pelvis, and mammography were negative. As possibility of choroidal metastasis could not be completely excluded based upon clinical examination, a diagnostic transvitreal FNAB was performed (**b**). Note biopsy site (arrow), localized subretinal hemorrhage (black arrowhead) and pocket of preretinal hemorrhage (white arrowhead). FNAB determined the mass to be choroidal melanoma (**c**). Following brachytherapy with episcleral 1–25 plaque performed, the tumor has undergone regression. Over the next 4 years, there has been absence of local and distant metastasis.

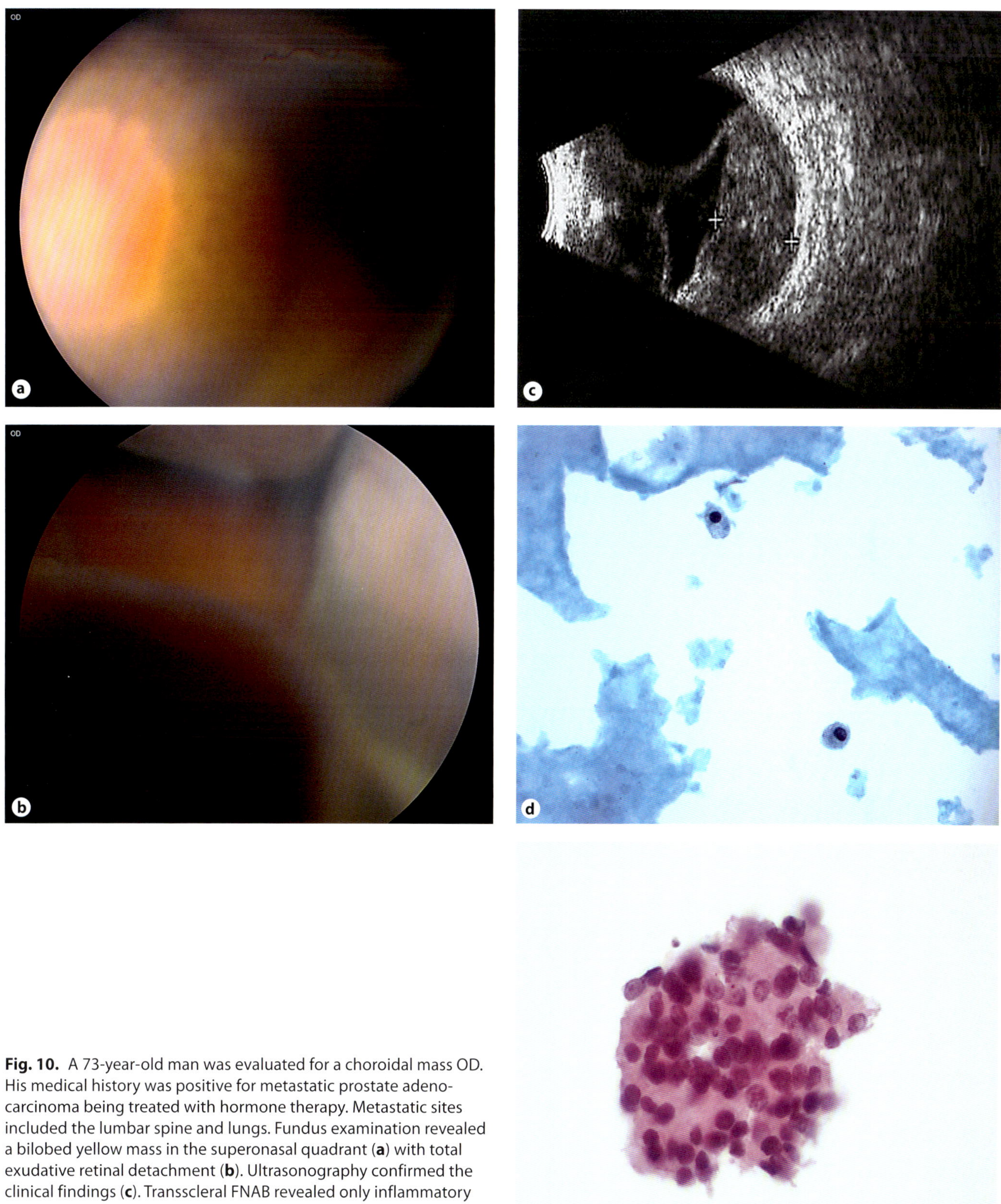

Fig. 10. A 73-year-old man was evaluated for a choroidal mass OD. His medical history was positive for metastatic prostate adenocarcinoma being treated with hormone therapy. Metastatic sites included the lumbar spine and lungs. Fundus examination revealed a bilobed yellow mass in the superonasal quadrant (**a**) with total exudative retinal detachment (**b**). Ultrasonography confirmed the clinical findings (**c**). Transscleral FNAB revealed only inflammatory cells with predominant histiocytes (**d**). Repeat FNAB was positive for adenocarcinoma (**e**).

References

1 Wickremasinghe S, Dansingani KK, Tranos P, Liyanage S, Jones A, Davey C: Ocular presentations of breast cancer. Acta Ophthalmol Scand 2007;85:133–142.

2 Weiss L: Analysis of the incidence of intraocular metastasis. Br J Ophthalmol 1993;77:149–151.

3 Shields CL, Shields JA, Gross NE, Schwartz GP, Lally SE: Survey of 520 eyes with uveal metastases. Ophthalmology 1997;104:1265–1276.

4 Soysal HG: Metastatic tumors of the uvea in 38 eyes. Can J Ophthalmol 2007;42:832–835.

5 Shields JA, Shields CL, Kiratli H, de Potter P: Metastatic tumors to the iris in 40 patients. Am J Ophthalmol 1995;119:422–430.

6 Lam A, Shields CL, Shields JA: Uveal metastases from breast carcinoma in three male patients. Ophthalmic Surg Lasers Imaging 2006;37:320–323.

7 Kreusel KM, Bechrakis NE, Wiegel T, Krause L, Foerster MH: Incidence and clinical characteristics of symptomatic choroidal metastasis from lung cancer. Acta Ophthalmol 2008;86:515–519.

8 Bandyopadhyay S, Adrean SD, Puklin JE, Feng J: Choroidal metastasis from an occult primary diagnosed by fine-needle aspiration: a case report. Diagn Cytopathol 2009;37:38–41.

9 Trichopoulos N, Augsburger JJ: Neuroendocrine tumours metastatic to the uvea: diagnosis by fine needle aspiration biopsy. Graefes Arch Clin Exp Ophthalmol 2006;244:524–528.

10 John VJ, Jacobson MS, Grossniklaus HE: Bilateral choroidal metastasis as the presenting sign of small cell lung carcinoma. J Thorac Oncol 2010;5:1289.

11 Van de Wouw AJ, Jansen RL, Speel EJ, Hillen HF: The unknown biology of the unknown primary tumour: a literature review. Ann Oncol 2003;14:191–196.

12 Kreusel KM, Bechrakis NE, Krause L, Wiegel T, Foerster MH: Incidence and clinical characteristics of symptomatic choroidal metastasis from breast cancer. Acta Ophthalmol Scand 2007;85:298–302.

13 Shome D, Honavar SG, Gupta P, Vemuganti GK, Reddy PV: Metastasis to the eye and orbit from renal cell carcinoma – a report of three cases and review of literature. Surv Ophthalmol 2007;52:213–223.

14 Shields JA, Shields CL, Ehya H, Eagle RC Jr, De Potter P: Fine-needle aspiration biopsy of suspected intraocular tumors: the 1992 Urwick lecture. Ophthalmology 1993;100:1677–1684.

15 Shields CL, Manquez ME, Ehya H, Mashayekhi A, Danzig CJ, Shields JA: Fine-needle aspiration biopsy of iris tumors in 100 consecutive cases: technique and complications. Ophthalmology 2006;113:2080–2086.

16 Augsburger JJ: Fine needle aspiration biopsy of suspected metastatic cancers to the posterior uvea. Trans Am Ophthalmol Soc 1988;86:499–560.

17 Kanthan GL, Jayamohan J, Yip D, Conway RM: Management of metastatic carcinoma of the uveal tract: an evidence-based analysis. Clin Experiment Ophthalmol 2007;35:553–565.

18 Baker S, Singh A, Tubbs R, Biscotti C: Uveal melanoma: an analysis of cellular features and comparison to monosomy 3 status. Cancer Cytopathol 2009;117:365.

19 Augsburger JJ, Shields JA, Folberg R, Lang W, O'Hara BJ, Claricci JD: Fine needle aspiration biopsy in the diagnosis of intraocular cancer: cytologic-histologic correlations. Ophthalmology 1985;92:39–49.

20 Schalenbourg A, Uffer S, Zografos L: Utility of a biopsy in suspicious pigmented iris tumors. Ophthalmic Res 2008;40:267–272.

21 Wesolowski R, Chung JY-H, Singh A, Kim R: Hepatocellular carcinoma metastatic to uvea. Retin Cases Brief Rep 2010;4:178–180.

22 Hood CT, Budd GT, Zakov ZN, Singh AD: Male breast carcinoma metastatic to the choroid: report of 3 cases and review of the literature. Eur J Ophthalmol 2010, E-pub ahead of print.

23 Pelayes D, Biscotti CV, Singh AD: Fine needle aspiration biopsy of an intraocular tumor. Vision Pan-America 2010;9:118–120.

24 Ylagan LR: Intraocular pigmented proliferations in the context of cytologic evaluation. Diagn Cytopathol 2009;37:853–864.

Arun D. Singh, MD, Professor of Ophthalmology
Director, Department of Ophthalmic Oncology, Cole Eye Institute, Cleveland Clinic Foundation
9500 Euclid Avenue
Cleveland, OH 44195 (USA)
Tel. +1 216 445 9479, E-Mail singha@ccf.org

Chapter 4

Biscotti CV, Singh AD (eds): FNA Cytology of Ophthalmic Tumors.
Monogr Clin Cytol. Basel, Karger 2012, vol 21, pp 31–43

Uveal Lymphoma

Deborah J. Chute[a] · Charles V. Biscotti[a] · Arun D. Singh[b]

Departments of [a]Anatomic Pathology and [b]Ophthalmology, Cleveland Clinic Foundation, Cleveland, Ohio, USA

Primary uveal lymphoma is rare and, unlike the vitreoretinal lymphomas, is typically indolent in nature [1–3]. In the past these tumors were termed 'reactive lymphoid hyperplasia' or 'uveal pseudotumor' because of their low-grade appearance [4–6]. However, convincing evidence with modern techniques has demonstrated that the majority of these lesions are low-grade B-cell lymphomas, most commonly extranodal marginal zone B-cell lymphomas [1, 5, 7] according to the current WHO classification (table 1) [8]. Primary high-grade lymphomas involving the uvea are extremely rare [26]. Uveal lymphoma may be considered primary if the uvea is the only or the initial site and secondary if there is secondary involvement of the uvea by systemic non-Hodgkin lymphoma [13, 27–34]. Hence, a careful clinical evaluation for involvement of other sites is required at the time of initial diagnosis and subsequent follow-up.

Etiology/Pathogenesis

The uvea does not contain normal lymphoid tissue, although this is not required for the development of an extranodal marginal zone B-cell lymphoma. The etiology of primary uveal lymphomas remains unknown.

Clinical Features

Choroidal lymphoma is typically unilateral, occurs more frequently in men than in women, and occurs more often in the 50–60s [1–3]. The most common presentation is recurrent, painless blurred vision and metamorphopsia due to retinal detachment. Other signs can include increased intraocular pressure, which can become painful. Proptosis can occur when extraocular involvement occurs, and if extending into the subconjunctival or episcleral regions, 'salmon patches' may be present [1, 2, 35–38].

On funduscopic examination, multifocal, yellow-pink choroidal infiltration occurs early (fig. 1a), followed by diffuse thickening of the uveal tract in late disease (fig. 1b). The vitreous fluid typically remains clear. Ancillary studies such as fluorescein angiography, indocyanine angiography (fig. 1c), optical coherence tomography (fig. 1d) and ultrasonography (fig. 1e) are essential in detecting subclinical involvement.

The differential diagnosis of primary uveal lymphoma includes both benign and malignant conditions such as choroidal hemangioma, posterior scleritis, uveal effusion syndrome, sarcoidosis and infectious agents, while metastasis and amelanotic melanoma must also be excluded [2, 3, 35, 37, 39–42].

Diagnostic Evaluation

Technique

Obtaining adequate, viable tissue for the diagnosis of primary uveal lymphoma can be difficult. The task becomes easy if concomitant adnexal involvement is detected (fig. 1e). Many different techniques are available, including transvitreal fine needle aspiration (FNA) and transscleral FNA. Chorioretinal biopsy is another option

Table 1. The current WHO classification of lymphomas [8]

- Hodgkin lymphoma
  - Nodular lymphocyte-predominant Hodgkin lymphoma
  - Classical Hodgkin lymphoma
- Non-Hodgkin lymphomas
  - B-cell lymphomas
    - Small cell lymphomas
      - Chronic lymphocytic leukemia/small lymphocytic lymphoma[1] [9, 10]
      - Extranodal marginal zone lymphoma[2] [1]
      - Follicular lymphoma[1] [11, 12]
      - Hairy cell leukemia
      - Lymphoplasmacytic lymphoma
      - Mantle cell lymphoma[1] [13, 14]
      - Nodal marginal zone lymphoma
      - Splenic marginal zone lymphoma
    - Large cell lymphomas
      - Burkitt lymphoma[1] [15–17]
      - Diffuse large B-cell lymphoma[2] [3, 18]
      - Intravascular large B-cell lymphoma[1] [19]
      - Lymphomatoid granulomatosis
      - Mediastinal (thymic) large B-cell lymphoma
      - Primary effusion lymphoma
    - Plasma cell neoplasms[1] [20, 21]
  - T-cell lymphomas
    - Adult T-cell leukemia/lymphoma[1] [22, 23]
    - Aggressive NK cell leukemia
    - Anaplastic large cell lymphoma[1] [24]
    - Angioimmunoblastic T-cell lymphoma
    - Enteropathy-type T-cell lymphoma
    - Extranodal NK/T-cell lymphoma[1] [24]
    - Hepatosplenic T-cell lymphoma
    - Mycosis fungoides[1] [25]
    - Peripheral T-cell lymphoma, unspecified[1, 2] [24]
    - Subcutaneous panniculitis-like T-cell lymphoma
    - Primary cutaneous CD30-positive T-cell lymphoproliferative disorders (e.g. lymphomatoid papulosis)

NK = Natural killer.
[1] Reported to secondarily involve the orbit or eye.
[2] Can occur as a primary intraocular or uveal lymphoma.

for obtaining tissue for analysis [Chapter 1, this vol., pp. 1–9] [43–45].

Sample Handling

Regardless of the biopsy method, it is critically important to work closely with the cytopathologist to ensure that tissue is collected and triaged appropriately. The cytopathologist must be made aware that lymphoma is in the differential diagnosis so that a portion of the sample can be set aside for special studies. In addition, the biopsy should be transported rapidly to the laboratory for evaluation. Lymphoma cells are fragile and can quickly degrade, resulting in a non-diagnostic specimen [2].

Cytological material can be kept undiluted or rinsed into a tissue medium solution such as Roswell Park Memorial Institute 1640 (Invitrogen, Carlsbad, Calif., USA), which maintains cell viability. The specimen should be refrigerated while awaiting transportation to maintain cell viability. However, if there is a prolonged delay in transportation, then an appropriate preservative should be used (e.g. Cytolyt, Cytyc Corp., Boxborough, Mass., USA). This will maintain cell morphology for cytological evaluation and allow immunohistochemical stains for further analysis, but precludes flow-cytometric analysis.

Sample Processing

Once the specimen has arrived in the cytology laboratory, a portion will be processed for cytological evaluation. The cells can be centrifuged into a pellet and the supernatant removed for interleukin studies if clinically requested (see below). If the processing laboratory does not perform interleukin testing, the supernatant can be frozen and held for processing at another laboratory. By centrifuging the sample, the number of cells available for cytological interpretation is maximized. A second portion of the sample can be set aside in a refrigerator, and triaged for special studies once an initial cytological impression confirms the presence of lymphocytes.

Cytological Evaluation

The sample can be processed by centrifugation to concentrate cells on a slide; this technique is called a cytospin and can then be stained using either a Papanicolaou or modified Wright-Giemsa stain. Alternatively, the sample can be processed using a Thinprep processor, which deposits cells on a thin membrane using vacuum, rather than centrifugation. The Thinprep slide can then be stained using the Papanicolaou method. Evaluation of the specimen for

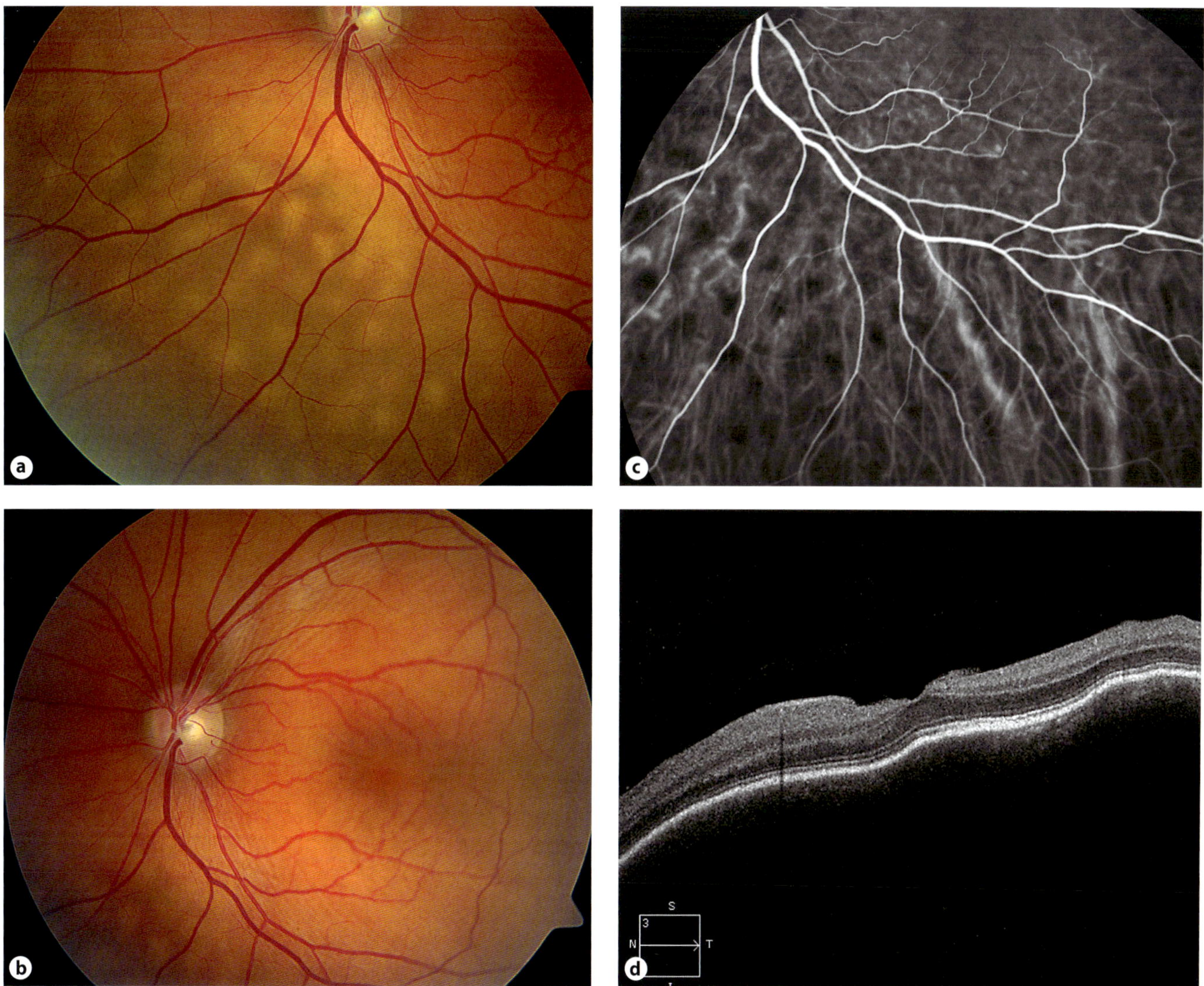

Fig. 1. A 48-year-old male presented with fluctuating vision in the left eye for the past 2 years. Prior ophthalmic examinations were reportedly normal. His medical history was remarkable only for hypertension and he had a negative oncological history. Ocular examination of the right eye was normal. The corrected visual acuity was 20/20–2 in the left eye. On external examination, 2 mm of proptosis was present. The left fundus examination revealed diffuse choroidal thickening (**a**) with focal choroidal infiltrates (**b**). Indocyanine green angiography was obtained and demonstrated hypofluorescent areas corresponding to areas of choroidal infiltrate (**c**). Optical coherence tomography showed irregular displacement of the retinal pigment epithelium with foveal distortion (**d**).

a monotonous population of lymphocytes with or without atypia can then be performed.

The cytomorphological appearance of uveal lymphomas is greatly dependent on the type of lymphoma present. As stated previously, lymphoma cells can be very fragile, and prompt transportation to the cytology laboratory is important to prevent cellular degeneration (fig. 2). A careful morphological examination is important, because malignant cells may be rare.

The most common primary uveal lymphoma, extranodal marginal zone lymphoma, is a low-grade indolent lymphoma comprised of small lymphocytes, centrocyte-like cells and a variable number of plasmacytoid cells. On Papanicolaou-stained slides, the cells are small with a relatively monomorphous appearance with scant cytoplasm and indistinct nucleoli (fig. 3). Diff-Quik staining artifactually gives the cells a larger appearance with more abundant cytoplasm, but the cells retain a monomorphous appearance with small, inconspicuous

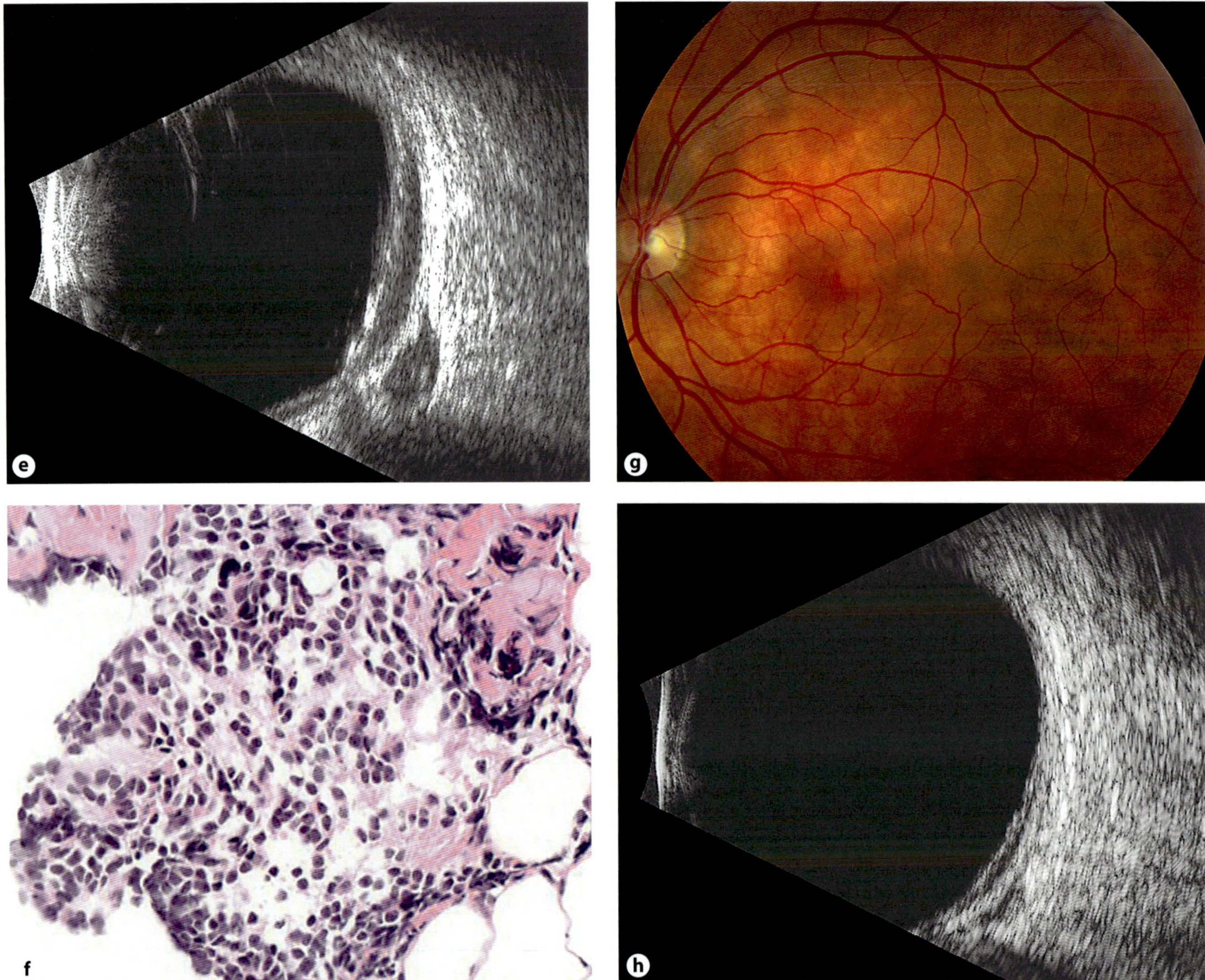

Fig. 1. Ultrasonography of the left eye revealed choroidal thickening with maximum elevation of 2.8 mm and an additional 3-mm orbital lesion temporal to the insertion of the optic nerve (**e**). Systemic evaluation including CT scans excluded suspicious lesions in the chest, abdomen and pelvis. Transconjunctival biopsy of the left orbit lesion was performed, and a fresh frozen section revealed lymphoid tissue. Biopsy and flow cytometry results demonstrated a monotypic λ small B-cell lymphocytic infiltrate consistent with mucosa-associated lymphoid tissue lymphoma (**f**). B cells were CD19, CD20 and CD45 positive, and CD4 negative. In the absence of lymphoma elsewhere, a final diagnosis of primary uveal lymphoma was made. Therapeutic options including low-dose radiation therapy versus targeted therapy with rituximab was discussed. Treatment with intravenous rituximab 375 mg/m^2 weekly for 4 weeks led to regression of the uveal (**g**) and extrascleral component (**h**).

nucleoli (fig. 4). In comparison, a reactive lymphoid proliferation can be similar but is often more polymorphous, with small lymphocytes and larger reactive centrocytes and immunoblasts (fig. 5). Because of the difficulty in distinguishing reactive lymphoid infiltrates from low-grade lymphomas, ancillary studies are required for definitive diagnosis.

On histological sections, extranodal marginal zone lymphoma of the uvea shows diffuse lymphocytic infiltration of the choroid, with or without involvement of the ciliary body (fig. 6a). Infiltration into the retinal pigment epithelium can occur. Follicles are frequently present, with surrounding expanded marginal zones and follicular colonization of the germinal centers, but these features may not be seen in small FNA biopsies. Immunohistochemistry will demonstrate a predominance of CD20-positive B cells (fig. 6b, c) with monotypic light chain restriction. Flow cytometry

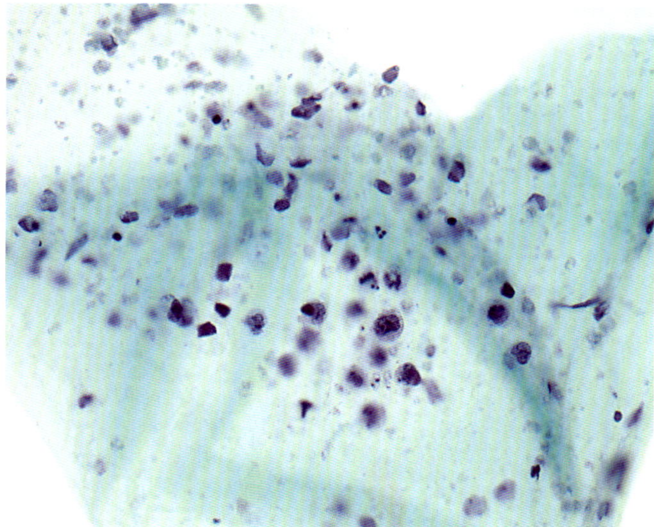

Fig. 2. Cytological preparation of a vitreous FNA demonstrating rare atypical cells, surrounded by extensive necrotic debris and degenerating cells; the final diagnosis was large cell lymphoma. Thinprep, Papanicolaou stain. ×400.

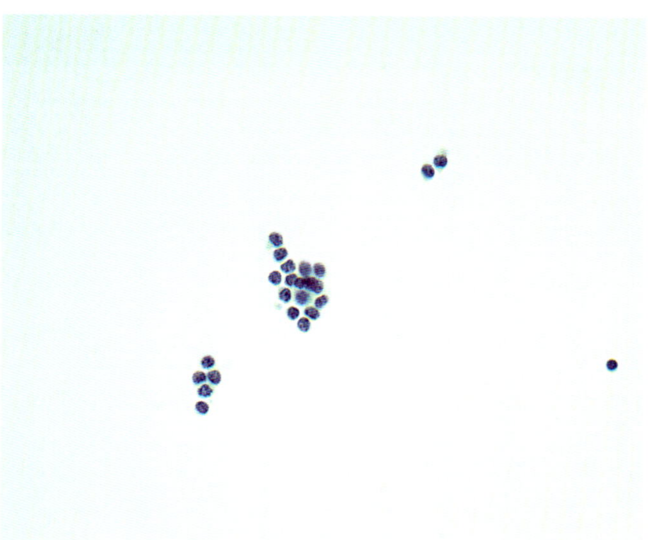

Fig. 3. Cytological preparation of choroidal eye FNA demonstrating small lymphocytes with minimal variation in size, coarse chromatin and inconspicuous nucleoli; the final diagnosis was extranodal marginal zone lymphoma. Thinprep, Papanicolaou stain. ×400.

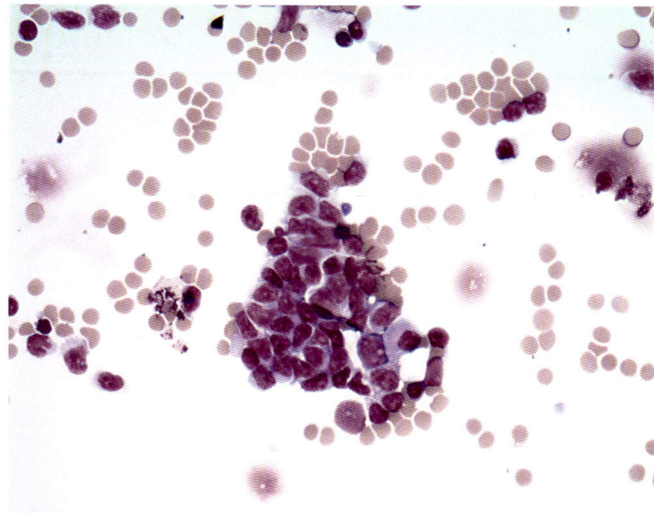

Fig. 4. Cytological preparation of choroidal eye FNA demonstrating small lymphocytes with more abundant cytoplasm and variation in size; the cytospin preparation can cause some distortion of cell size and shape due to the centrifugal forces used in sedimenting cells onto the slide – this is the same case as figure 3; the final diagnosis was extranodal marginal zone lymphoma. Cytospin, Diff-Quik stain. ×400.

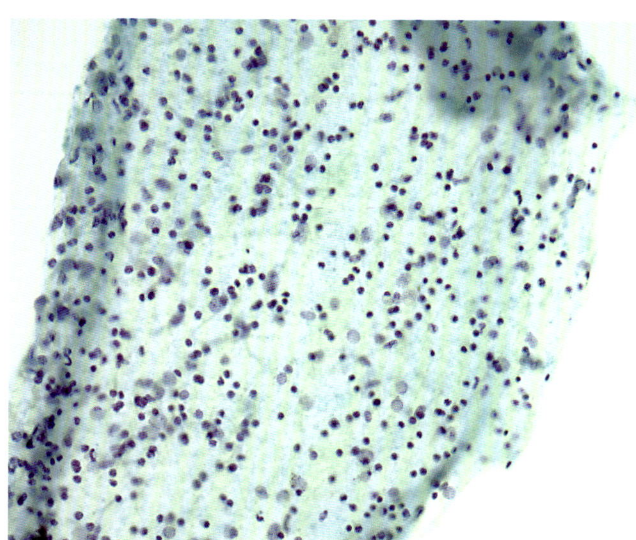

Fig. 5. Cytological preparation of vitreous fluid FNA with reactive population of lymphocytes; note the variation in cell size with multiple small lymphocytes and scattered larger centrocytes and immunoblasts. Flow cytometry on this case was negative for a lymphoproliferative disorder. Thinprep, Papanicolaou stain. ×200.

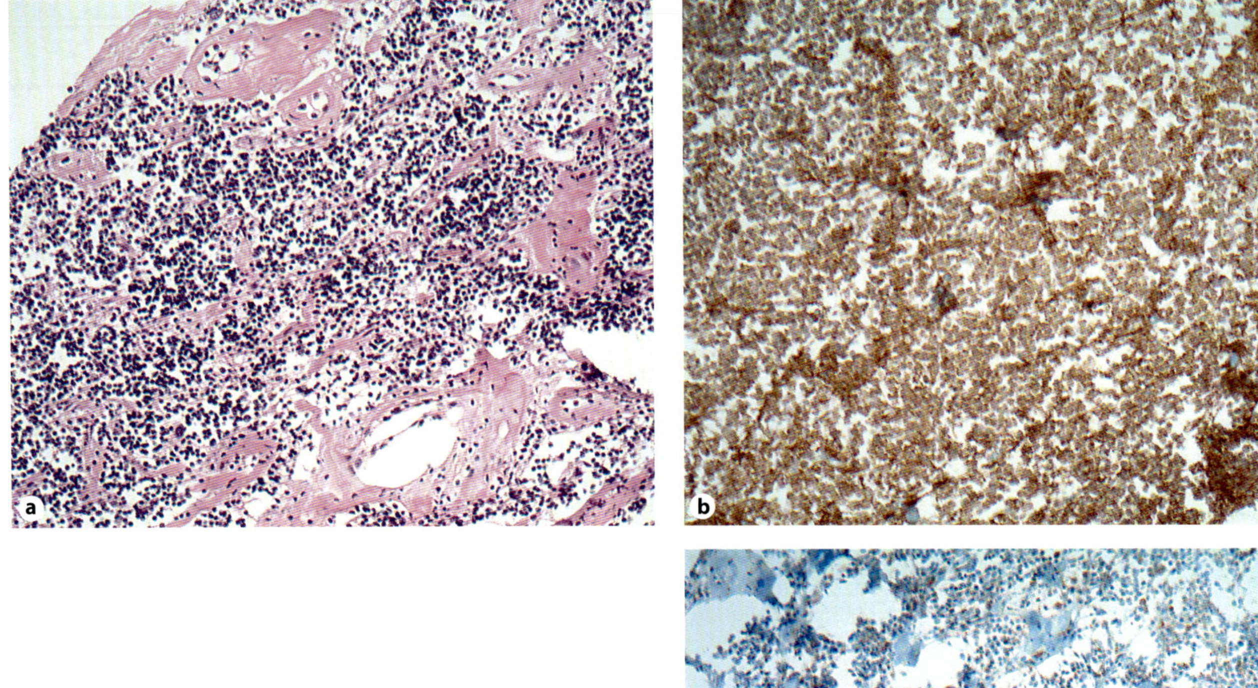

Fig. 6. Surgical biopsy of a uveal extranodal marginal zone lymphoma demonstrating diffuse infiltration of the sclera and adjacent fat by a monotonous population of small lymphocytes with minimal variation in size or shape (**a**, hematoxylin-eosin. ×200). Immunohistochemical staining with CD20 demonstrates all lymphocytes are B cells (**b**, CD20. ×200). CD3 is negative confirming the absence of T cells (**c**, CD3. ×200).

demonstrates a B-cell population that is (κ/λ) light chain restricted (fig. 7).

Large cell lymphoma can rarely be primary to the uvea but is much more likely the intraocular extension of systemic disease or uveal involvement from a primary vitreous/retinal lymphoma. In this setting, cytology demonstrates a monotonous population of large atypical lymphocytes with large nuclei and prominent nucleoli (fig. 8). A diagnosis of malignant lymphoma is easily established by cytology in this setting, but ancillary testing may be used for further subtyping.

Uveal involvement of other systemic lymphomas can occur, and the cytological appearance can be highly variable, depending on the type of non-Hodgkin lymphoma (fig. 9–13).

Ancillary Studies

Immunohistochemistry

Although cytological diagnosis is the gold standard in the diagnosis of intraocular lymphoma, immunohistochemistry can be very helpful for confirmation and classification according to the WHO's system. B-cell and T-cell lymphocytes express different surface antigens, which allow differentiation between lymphoma subtypes (table 2) [46, 47].

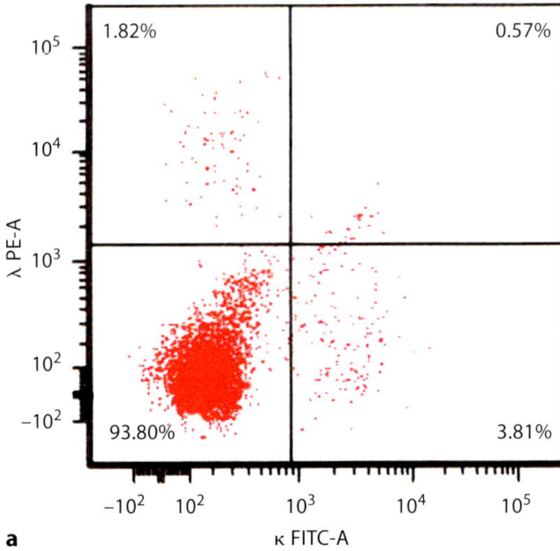

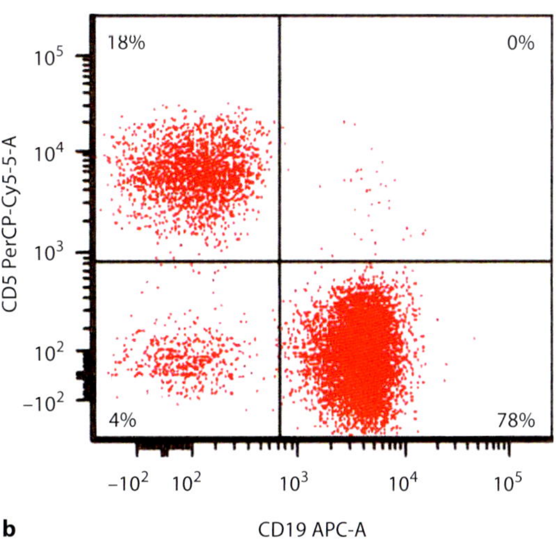

Fig. 7. Flow cytometry dot plot demonstrating a normal κ-to-λ ratio. B cells positive for λ light chains are present in the upper left corner, B cells positive for κ light chains are present in the lower right corner, and T cells which express neither marker are present in the lower left corner. In this case, the κ-to-λ ratio is 3.8 to 1.8, or 2:1 (**a**). Flow cytometry dot plot demonstrating a large B-cell population in the sample. CD19 is a marker of B cells and CD5 is a marker of T cells, so B cells are present in the right corner comprising 78% of all cells. In this case, there is no aberrant coexpression of CD19 and CD5 on the B cells (**b**). Flow cytometry dot plot from the same case as in **b** showing a large κ-light-chain-restricted population of B cells, present in the lower right corner; the κ-to-λ ratio in this case is 72:1 (**c**).

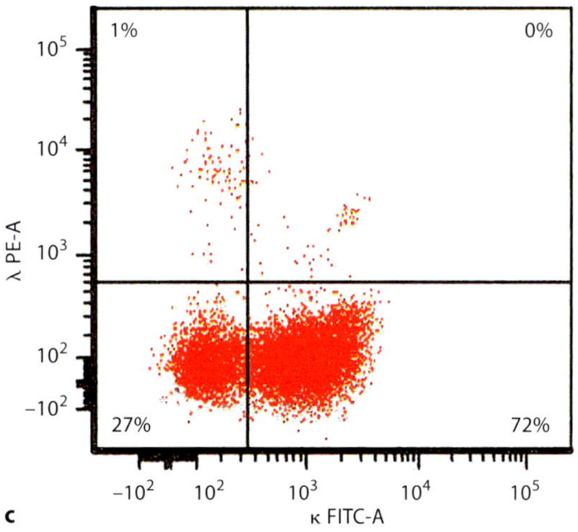

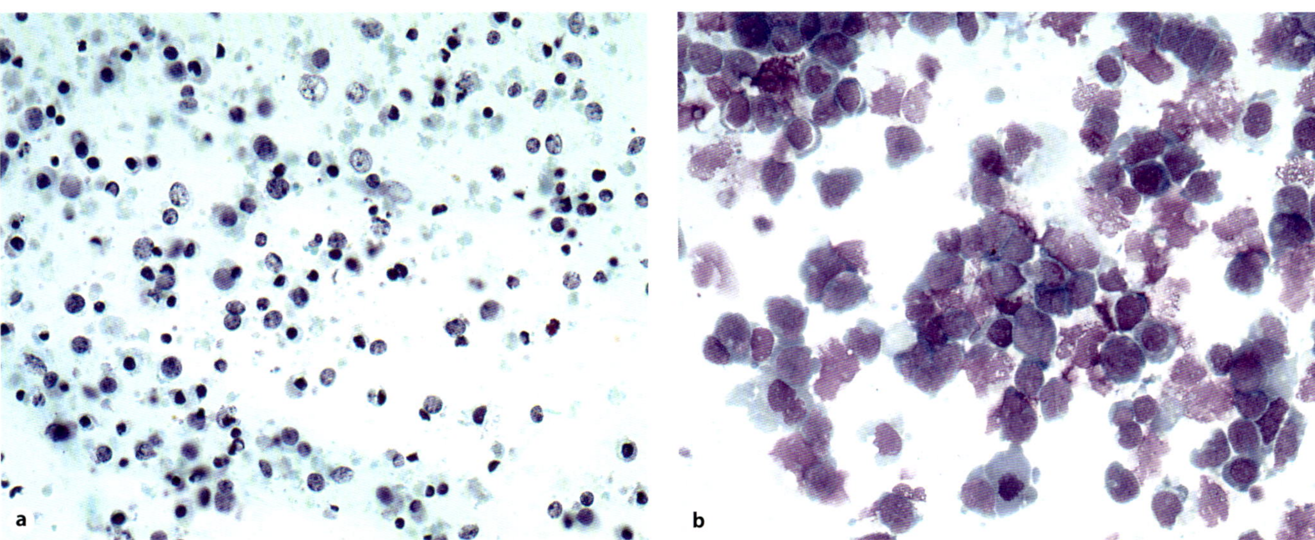

Fig. 8. Large B-cell lymphoma. Cytological preparation of a vitrectomy sample demonstrating large, atypical lymphoid cells with prominent nucleoli in a background of apoptosis and necrotic debris (**a**, Thinprep, Papanicolaou stain. ×400). Note atypical lymphocytes with irregular nuclear contours, marked pleomorphism and prominent nucleoli (**b**, Cytospin, Diff-Quik stain. ×400).

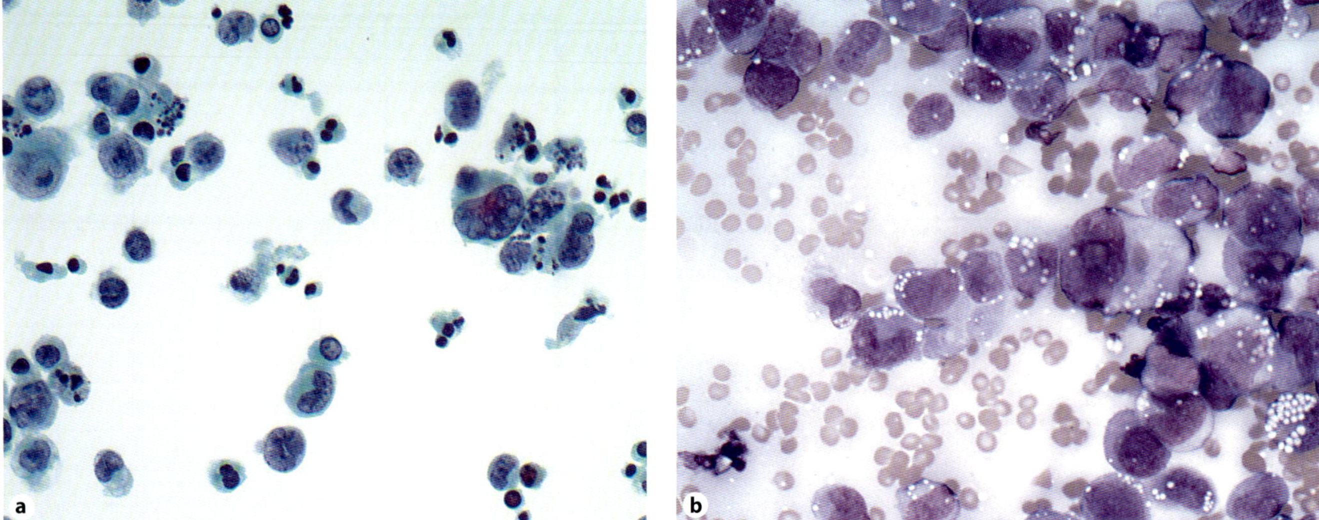

Fig. 9. Cytological preparation of anaplastic large cell lymphoma showing markedly enlarged cells, extensive pleomorphism and classic 'horseshoe-shaped' nuclei; this patient was originally diagnosed with anaplastic large cell lymphoma in an inguinal lymph node FNA. (**a**, Thinprep, Papanicolaou stain, ×400) (**b**, FNA smear, Diff-Quik stain. ×400).

Evaluation of κ and λ light chain expression will determine B-cell monoclonality, a feature of most B-cell lymphomas. In a reactive population, the κ-to-λ ratio should be near 2:1 due to random selection, but in a B-cell lymphoma, all of the cells will express the same light chain [8]. Therefore, a predominance of one light chain is suggestive of a B-cell lymphoma. Unfortunately, a similar marker of T-cell clonality is not available by immunohistochemistry, and molecular testing is often required for the diagnosis of T-cell lymphomas. Immunohistochemistry can be performed on thin-layer cytology slides and cell blocks, as well as on formalin-fixed tissue biopsies. A limitation of this technique is that each immunohistochemical stain requires an additional slide for evaluation.

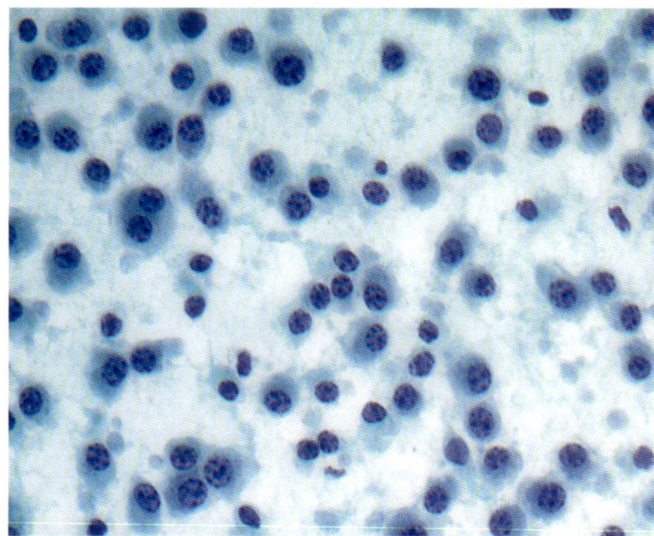

Fig. 10. Cytological preparation of plasma cell myeloma showing lymphoid cells with eccentric, plasmacytoid cytoplasm and round nuclei with coarse, 'clock face' chromatin; this patient was originally diagnosed with plasma cell myeloma in a bone marrow biopsy. FNA smear, Papanicolaou stain. ×400.

Flow Cytometry

Flow cytometry is a very powerful tool in the diagnosis of lymphoma, but it requires viable cells in suspension [48–50]. This technique uses antibodies similar to immunohistochemistry but can analyze multiple different markers simultaneously on the lymphoma cells, including κ and λ light chains (fig. 7). Flow cytometry is particularly helpful in cases with limited material, which is a common problem with intraocular lymphomas. However, if many reactive lymphocytes are present, the lymphoma signal can be lost in the background. In one study of intraocular lymphomas,

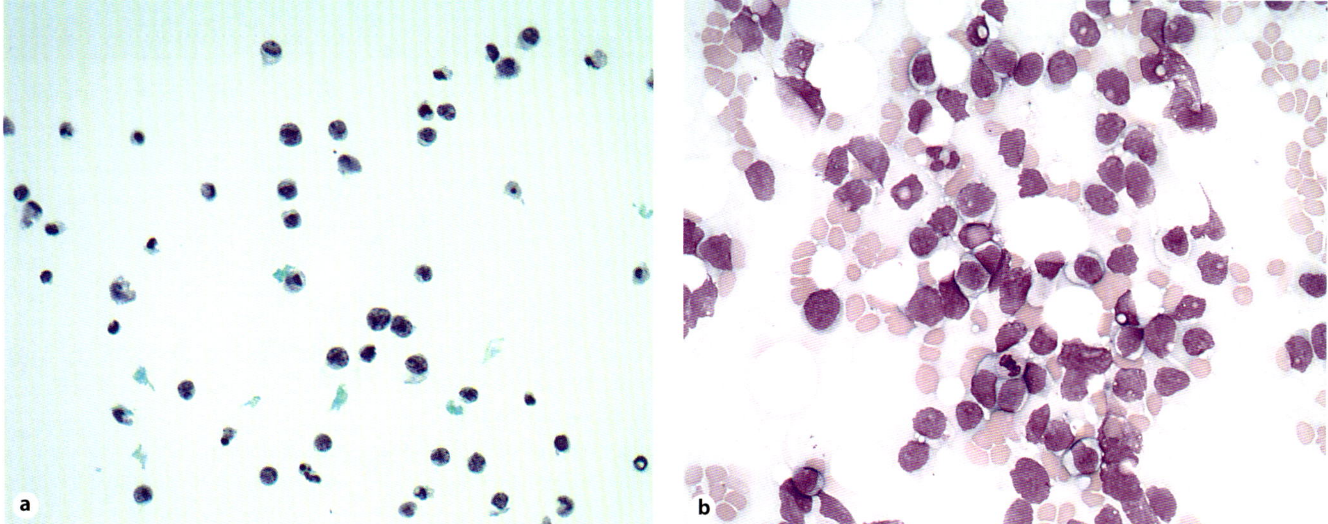

Fig. 11. Cytological preparation of an anterior chamber aqueous aspirate demonstrating intermediate size lymphocytes with irregular nuclear contours and a moderate amount of cytoplasm; the final diagnosis was involvement by mantle cell lymphoma which had previously been diagnosed in a lymph node (**a**, ThinPrep, Papanicolaou stain. ×400). A different patient's uveal FNA also shows intermediate size lymphocytes with fine chromatin, irregular nuclear contours and variably sized nucleoli; the final diagnosis was blastic variant of mantle cell lymphoma (**b**, FNA smear, Diff-Quik stain. ×400).

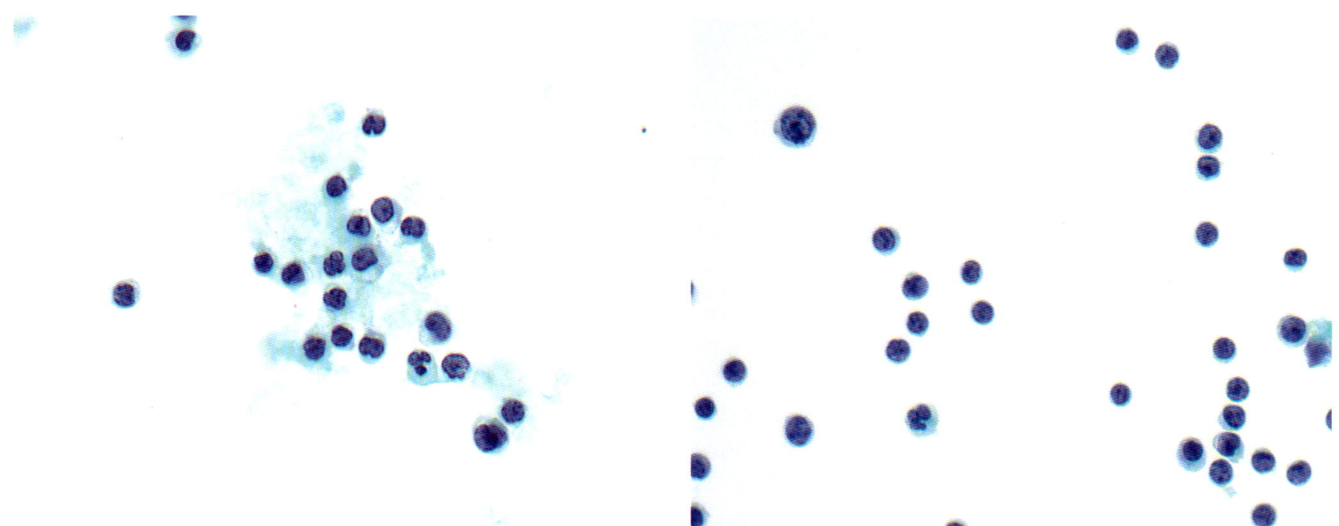

Fig. 12. Cytological preparation of adult T-cell lymphoma/leukemia demonstrating intermediate size lymphocytes with the classic 4-lobed nuclei (shamrock-like); this patient was originally diagnosed with adult T-cell lymphoma involving the peripheral blood and pleural fluid. Thinprep, Papanicolaou stain. ×400.

Fig. 13. Cytological preparation of peripheral T-cell lymphoma not otherwise specified, demonstrating a monotonous population of intermediate to large atypical lymphocytes with irregular nuclear contours and prominent nucleoli; this patient was originally diagnosed with peripheral T-cell lymphoma not otherwise specified in a pleural effusion sample. Thinprep, Papanicolaou stain. ×400.

Table 2. Immunohistochemical markers for the diagnosis of lymphoma

Marker	B-cell lineage	T-cell lineage	Comment
CD45	+	+	General marker of lymphoid tissue
CD20	+	–	May be lost after rituximab (anti-CD20) therapy
CD19	+	–	
CD79a[1]	+	–	
Pax5[1]	+	–	
CD3	–	+	
CD5	–	+	Can be aberrantly expressed in some B-cell lymphomas (e.g. CLL, MCL)
CD7	–	+	Loss of CD7 is the most common abnormality in T-cell lymphomas
CD56	–	+/–	Natural killer cell marker
CD23	+/–	–	Aberrantly expressed in CLL
CD10	+/–	–	Marker of germinal center cells; positive in FL and some DLBCL
κ light chain	+	–	Used in conjunction with λ light chain to determine monoclonality for B cells
λ light chain	+	–	Used in conjunction with κ light chain to determine monoclonality for B cells
BCL-2[1]	+	–	Overexpressed in FL due to t(14;18) translocation and some DLBCL
Cyclin D1[1]	+/–	–	Overexpressed in MCL due to t(11;14) translocation
CD138	+/–	–	Marker of plasmacytic differentiation
CD34	–	–	Marker of immature myeloid cells (myeloid leukemia)

CLL = Chronic lymphocytic leukemia; MCL = mantle cell lymphoma; DLBCL = diffuse large B-cell lymphoma; FL = follicular lymphoma.
[1] These markers are not available for flow cytometry.

flow cytometry was helpful in making the diagnosis in 7 out of 10 cases [51].

Molecular Testing

In difficult cases, molecular testing may be used to confirm the presence of lymphoma. [52–54] This is most commonly performed by looking for clonal rearrangements of the heavy chain of the immunoglobulin gene (IgH; B-cell clonality) or the γ-chain of the T-cell receptor (T-cell clonality). DNA is extracted from fresh or fixed lymphocytes, and polymerase chain reaction (PCR) is performed using primers specific for the genetic area of interest. A reactive lymphoid proliferation will show a diffuse band of PCR products, while lymphoma samples will show a single discrete PCR product (fig. 14).

Advances in our understanding of lymphoma have resulted in recognition of a number of recurring genetic abnormalities in certain lymphoma subtypes [8]. The presence or absence of these translocations and genetic deletions can be identified using fluorescence in situ hybridization (FISH), immunohistochemistry and/or PCR (table 3). FISH is particularly useful in cytological specimens, as only a few lymphoma cells are needed to perform hybridization and evaluation (fig. 15) [55]. In patients with a known systemic non-Hodgkin lymphoma, FISH analysis may provide rapid identification of intraocular involvement.

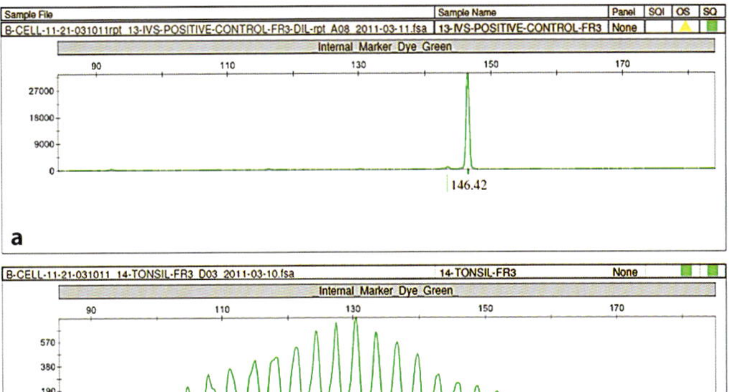

Fig. 14. Lymphoid samples can be tested for clonality using molecular techniques, such as immunoglobulin heavy chain (IgH) rearrangements. In a nonneoplastic lymphoid population (e.g. normal tonsil tissue), all of the B lymphocytes will have IgH PCR products of slightly different lengths. Depending on how the result is analyzed, this results in a broad band (gel electrophoresis) or multiple peaks (capillary electrophoresis). However, all of the cells in a B-cell lymphoma will have IgH PCR products of identical length, resulting in a single band or single peak. This figure compares the products from an IgH PCR reaction run on capillary electrophoresis for a B-cell lymphoma demonstrating a single large peak (**a**) versus a reactive tonsil demonstrating multiple peaks (**b**).

Table 3. Recurring genetic abnormalities in lymphomas [8]

Diagnosis	Genetic abnormality	Frequency %
Small lymphocytic lymphoma/ chronic lymphocytic leukemia	del(11q22–23) – poor prognosis del(13q14) – better prognosis	18 55
Mantle cell lymphoma	t(11;14)(q13;q32) *CCND1-IGH*	>95
Marginal zone lymphoma	t(11;14)(q21;132) *MALT1-IGH*	25–50
Follicular lymphoma	t(14;18)(q32;q21) *IGH-BCL2*	70–95
Burkitt's lymphoma	t(8;14)(q24;32) *MYC-IGH*	85
Anaplastic large cell lymphoma	t(2;5)(p23;q35) *NPM1-ALK*	70–80
Diffuse large B-cell lymphoma	Germinal center type *(GCB)* t(14;18), CD10 and BCL-6 expression; better prognosis	40
	Activated B-cell type gain chromosome 3, *MUM1* expression; worse prognosis	34

del = Deletion.

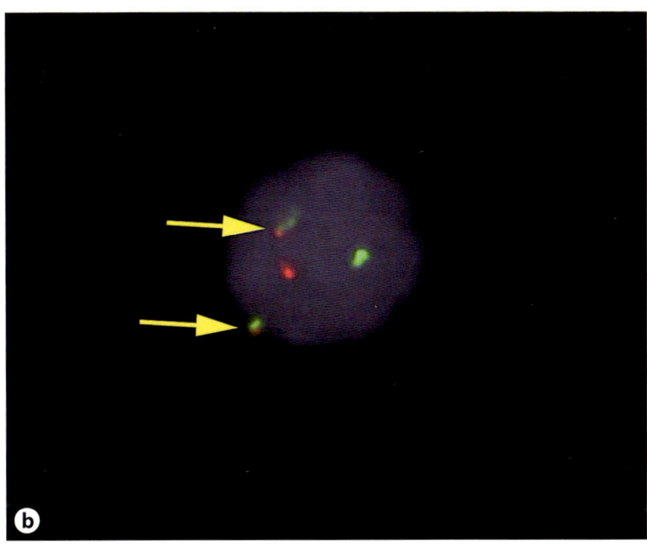

Fig. 15. FISH testing for the t(11;14) translocation found in mantle cell lymphoma. Two fluorescently labeled probes, one for chromosome 11 near the *CCND1* gene and one for chromosome 14 near the *IGH* gene, are hybridized to a thin layer of lesional cells. A negative result will show 2 discrete green and 2 discrete red signals in each cell nucleus. FISH t(11;14) (**a**, x 400). A positive result will show 2 areas with green and red signals adjacent to each other (in some situations resulting in a yellow fusion signal; yellow arrows point to fusion signals), consistent with the presence of a translocation. FISH t(11;14) (**b**, × 400).

References

1 Coupland SE, Foss HD, Hidayat AA, Cockerham GC, Hummel M, Stein H: Extranodal marginal zone B cell lymphomas of the uvea: an analysis of 13 cases. J Pathol 2002;197:333–340.

2 Coupland SE, Damato B: Understanding intraocular lymphomas. Clin Experiment Ophthalmol 2008;36:564–578.

3 Coupland SE, Heimann H, Bechrakis NE: Primary intraocular lymphoma: a review of the clinical, histopathological and molecular biological features. Graefes Arch Clin Exp Ophthalmol 2004;242:901–913.

4 Ryan SJ, Zimmerman LE, King FM: Reactive lymphoid hyperplasia: an unusual form of intraocular pseudotumor. Trans Am Acad Ophthalmol Otolaryngol 1972;76:652–671.

5 Cockerham GC, Hidayat AA, Bijwaard KE, Sheng ZM: Re-evaluation of 'reactive lymphoid hyperplasia of the uvea': an immunohistochemical and molecular analysis of 10 cases. Ophthalmology 2000;107:151–158.

6 Crookes GP, Mullaney J: Lymphoid hyperplasia of the uveal tract simulating malignant lymphoma. Am J Ophthalmol 1967;63:962–967.

7 Ben-Ezra D, Sahel JA, Harris NL, Hemo I, Albert DM: Uveal lymphoid infiltrates: immunohistochemical evidence for a lymphoid neoplasia. Br J Ophthalmol 1989;73:846–851.

8 Jaffe ES, Harris NL, Stein H, Vardiman JW (eds): World Health Organization Classification of Tumors: Tumors of Haematopoietic and Lymphoid Tissue. Lyons; IARC Press, 2001.

9 Coupland SE, Foss HD, Bechrakis NE, Hummel M, Stein H: Secondary ocular involvement in systemic 'memory' B-cell lymphocytic leukemia. Ophthalmology 2001;108:1289–1295.

10 Ong YL, White S: Intra-vitreal methotrexate leads to resolution of intraocular chronic lymphocytic leukaemia. Br J Haematol 2010;148:181.

11 O'Keefe JS, Sippy BD, Martin DF, Holden JT, Grossniklaus HE: Anterior chamber infiltrates associated with systemic lymphoma: report of two cases and review of the literature. Ophthalmology 2002;109:253–257.

12 Stacy RC, Jakobiec FA, Schoenfield L, Singh AD: Unifocal and multifocal reactive lymphoid hyperplasia vs follicular lymphoma of the ocular adnexa. Am J Ophthalmol 2010;150:412–426.

13 Ahn ES, Singh AD, Smith SD: Mantle cell lymphoma with uveal metastasis. Leuk Lymphoma 2010;51:1354–1355.

14 Rowley SA, Fahy GT, Brown LJ: Mantle cell lymphoma presenting as a choroidal mass: part of the spectrum of uveal lymphoid infiltration. Eye (Lond) 2000;14:241–244.

15 Feman SS, Niwayama G, Hepler RS, Foos RY: 'Burkitt tumor' with intraocular involvement. Surv Ophthalmol 1969;14:106–111.

16 Payne T, Karp LA, Zimmerman LE: Intraocular involvement in Burkitt's lymphoma. Arch Ophthalmol 1971;85:295–298.

17 Wysenbeek YS, Nissenkorn I, Cohen S, Ben-Sira I, Stark B, Zaizov R: Intraocular involvement of Burkitt's lymphoma in a Bedouin child. Pediatr Hematol Oncol 1987;4:309–314.

18 Faia LJ, Chan CC. Primary intraocular lymphoma. Arch Pathol Lab Med 2009;133:1228–1232.

19 Mudhar HS, Sethuraman C, Khan MD, Jan SU: Intraocular, pan-uveal intravascular large B-cell lymphoma associated with choroidal infarction and choroidal tri-lineage extramedullary haemtopoiesis. Histopathology 2007;51:275–279.

20 Liu K, Klintworth GK, Dodd LG: Cytologic findings in vitreous fluids: analysis of 74 specimens. Acta Cytol 1999;43:201–206.

21 Shakin EP, Augsburger JJ, Eagle RC Jr, et al: Multiple myeloma involving the iris. Arch Ophthalmol 1988;106:524–526.

22 Kohno T, Uchida H, Inomata H, Fukushima S, Takeshita M, Kikuchi M: Ocular manifestations of adult T-cell leukemia/lymphoma: a clinicopathologic study. Ophthalmology 1993;100:1794–1799.

23 Kumar SR, Gill PS, Wagner DG, Dugel PU, Moudgil T, Rao NA: Human T-cell lymphotropic virus type I-associated retinal lymphoma: a clinicopathologic report. Arch Ophthalmol 1994;112:954–959.

24 Coupland SE, Foss HD, Assaf C, et al: T-cell and T/natural killer-cell lymphomas involving ocular and ocular adnexal tissues: a clinicopathologic, immunohistochemical, and molecular study of seven cases. Ophthalmology 1999;106:2109–2120.

25 Erny BC, Egbert PR, Peat IM, Shorrock K, Rosenthal AR: Intraocular involvement with subretinal pigment epithelium infiltrates by mycosis fungoides. Br J Ophthalmol 1991;75:698–701.

26 Shields JA, Shields CL: Intraocular Tumors: Atlas and Textbook. Philadelphia, Lippincott, Williams & Wilkins, 2008.

27 Fernandez-Suntay JP, Gragoudas ES, Ferry JA, Anderson ME, Dacey MP, Dryja TP: High-grade uveal B-cell lymphoma as the initial feature in Richter syndrome. Arch Ophthalmol 2002;120:1383–1385.

28 Shields JA, Shields CL, Scartozzi R: Survey of 1,264 patients with orbital tumors and simulating lesions: the 2002 Montgomery lecture. Part 1. Ophthalmology 2004;111:997–1008.

29 Mathai A, Lall A, Jain R, Pathengay A: Systemic non-Hodgkin's lymphoma masquerading as Vogt-Koyanagi-Harada disease in an HIV-positive patient. Clin Experiment Ophthalmol 2006;34:280–282.

30 Levy-Clarke GA, Greenman D, Sieving PC, et al: Ophthalmic manifestations, cytology, immunohistochemistry, and molecular analysis of intraocular metastatic T-cell lymphoma: report of a case and review of the literature. Surv Ophthalmol 2008;53:285–295.

31 Kiratli H, Bilgic S, Emec S: Simultaneous conjunctival, uveal, and orbital involvement as the initial sign of acute lymphoblastic leukemia. Jpn J Ophthalmol 2007;51:139–141.

32 Kase S, Saito W, Saito A, Ohno S: Uveal effusion syndrome caused by choroidal invasion of malignant lymphoma. Jpn J Ophthalmol 2010;54:109–110.

33 Fredrick DR, Char DH, Ljung BM, Brinton DA: Solitary intraocular lymphoma as an initial presentation of widespread disease. Arch Ophthalmol 1989;107:395–397.

34 al-Hazzaa SA, Green WR, Mann RB: Uveal involvement in systemic angiotropic large cell lymphoma: microscopic and immunohistochemical studies. Ophthalmology 1993;100:961–965.

35 Rasic DM, Stankovic Z, Terzic T, Kovacevic D, Koturovic Z, Markovic V: Primary extranodal marginal zone lymphoma of the uvea associated with massive diffuse epibulbar extension and focal infiltration of the optic nerve and meninges, clinically presented as uveitis masquerade syndrome: a case report. Med Oncol 2010;27:1010–1016.

36 Ramulu P, Iliff NT, Green WR, Kuo IC: Asymptomatic conjunctival mucosa-associated lymphoid tissue-type lymphoma with presumed intraocular involvement. Cornea 2007;26:484–486.

37 Holz FG, Boehmer HV, Mechtersheimer G, Ott G, Volcker HE: Uveal non-Hodgkin's lymphoma with epibulbar extension simulating choroidal effusion syndrome. Retina 1999;19:343–346.

38 Cursiefen C, Holbach LM, Lafaut B, Heimann K, Kirchner T, Naumann GO: Oculocerebral non-Hodgkin's lymphoma with uveal involvement: development of an epibulbar tumor after vitrectomy. Arch Ophthalmol 2000;118:1437–1440.

39 Chang TS, Byrne SF, Gass JD, Hughes JR, Johnson RN, Murray TG. Echographic findings in benign reactive lymphoid hyperplasia of the choroid. Arch Ophthalmol 1996;114:669–675.

40 Jensen OA, Johansen S, Kiss K: Intraocular T-cell lymphoma mimicking a ring melanoma. First manifestation of systemic disease. Report of a case and survey of the literature. Graefes Arch Clin Exp Ophthalmol 1994;232:148–152.

41 Sen HN, Bodaghi B, Hoang PL, Nussenblatt R: Primary intraocular lymphoma: diagnosis and differential diagnosis. Ocul Immunol Inflamm 2009;17:133–141.

42 Tavallali A, Shields CL, Bianciotto C, Shields JA: Choroidal lymphoma masquerading as anterior ischemic optic neuropathy. Eur J Ophthalmol 2010;20:959–962.

43 Gonzales JA, Chan CC: Biopsy techniques and yields in diagnosing primary intraocular lymphoma. Int Ophthalmol 2007;27:241–250.

44 Coupland SE, Joussen A, Anastassiou G, Stein H: Diagnosis of a primary uveal extranodal marginal zone B-cell lymphoma by chorioretinal biopsy: case report. Graefes Arch Clin Exp Ophthalmol 2005;243:482–486.

45 Cole CJ, Kwan AS, Laidlaw DA, Aylward GW: A new technique of combined retinal and choroidal biopsy. Br J Ophthalmol 2008;92:1357–1360.

46 Davis JL, Solomon D, Nussenblatt RB, Palestine AG, Chan CC: Immunocytochemical staining of vitreous cells. Indications, techniques, and results. Ophthalmology 1992;99:250–256.

47 Wilson DJ, Braziel R, Rosenbaum JT: Intraocular lymphoma. Immunopathologic analysis of vitreous biopsy specimens. Arch Ophthalmol 1992; 110:1455–1458.

48 Demurtas A, Accinelli G, Pacchioni D, et al: Utility of flow cytometry immunophenotyping in fine-needle aspirate cytologic diagnosis of non-Hodgkin lymphoma: a series of 252 cases and review of the literature. Appl Immunohistochem Mol Morphol 2010;18:311–322.

49 Davis JL, Miller DM, Ruiz P: Diagnostic testing of vitrectomy specimens. Am J Ophthalmol 2005;140:822–829.

50 Zaldivar RA, Martin DF, Holden JT, Grossniklaus HE: Primary intraocular lymphoma: clinical, cytologic, and flow cytometric analysis. Ophthalmology 2004;111:1762–1767.

51 Davis JL, Viciana AL, Ruiz P: Diagnosis of intraocular lymphoma by flow cytometry. Am J Ophthalmol 1997;124:362–372.

52 Baehring JM, Androudi S, Longtine JJ, et al: Analysis of clonal immunoglobulin heavy chain rearrangements in ocular lymphoma. Cancer 2005;104:591–597.

53 Chan CC: Molecular pathology of primary intraocular lymphoma. Trans Am Ophthalmol Soc 2003;101:275–292.

54 Shen DF, Zhuang Z, LeHoang P, et al: Utility of microdissection and polymerase chain reaction for the detection of immunoglobulin gene rearrangement and translocation in primary intraocular lymphoma. Ophthalmology 1998;105:1664–1669.

55 Safley AM, Buckley PJ, Creager AJ, et al: The value of fluorescence in situ hybridization and polymerase chain reaction in the diagnosis of B-cell non-Hodgkin lymphoma by fine-needle aspiration. Arch Pathol Lab Med 2004;128:1395–1403.

Arun D. Singh, MD, Professor of Ophthalmology
Director, Department of Ophthalmic Oncology, Cole Eye Institute, Cleveland Clinic Foundation
9500 Euclid Avenue
Cleveland, OH 44195 (USA)
Tel. +1 216 445 9479, E-Mail singha@ccf.org

Biscotti CV, Singh AD (eds): FNA Cytology of Ophthalmic Tumors.
Monogr Clin Cytol. Basel, Karger 2012, vol 21, pp 44–54

Uveal Melanoma: Diagnostic Features

Charles V. Biscotti[a] · Arun D. Singh[b]

[a]Department of Anatomic Pathology and [b]Cole Eye Institute, Cleveland Clinic Foundation, Cleveland, Ohio, USA

Fine needle aspiration biopsy (FNAB) has widespread acceptance as an effective diagnostic test for uveal melanoma, albeit indicated in only a small minority of cases [1–3]. Clinical examination, including ophthalmoscopic evaluation, almost always establishes the diagnosis (fig. 1). For example only 2.5% of patients with ocular tumors required diagnostic FNAB in a large series [1]. This increased to 7% in a series of iris lesions [4]. FNAB is effective and indicated in the rare clinically ambiguous cases, especially those with melanoma and metastasis in the differential diagnosis. In fact approximately two thirds of all diagnostic ocular FNABs are performed to confirm a clinical impression of melanoma or metastasis [1].

Clinical Features

Melanomas are the most common primary uveal malignancy in adults. Uveal melanomas can also affect adolescents, children and neonates. Light-skinned people are at risk, and uveal melanoma rarely affects people of African or Asian descent. Uveal melanoma accounts for approximately 85% of ocular melanomas while approximately 15% arise in the conjunctiva [2]. Only approximately 2–5% arise in the iris [2, 5]. The remainder arise in the posterior uvea, mostly the choroid. Patients usually present with painless visual loss but can be asymptomatic [6].

Histology

Any discussion of uveal melanoma's cellular features benefits from understanding the histological features and classification. Callender [7] originally proposed a 6-tiered histological classification for uveal melanoma including: spindle A, spindle B, mixed cell, epithelioid cell, fascicular, and necrotic. Spindle A cells have a bland fusiform shape with uniform, narrow, oval nuclei containing inconspicuous nucleoli. Subsequently, most tumors that would have been classified as spindle A melanoma are now interpreted as nevi [8], and Callender's classification has been modified to a 3-tiered system: spindle cell melanoma, mixed cell melanoma and epithelioid cell melanoma [8]. The spindle cell type must be pure. No consensus exists regarding the percentage of epithelioid cells that distinguish the mixed cell type from the epithelioid one. Spindle cell melanoma cells have a fusiform or multipolar cytoplasmic shape and an oval or elongate nucleus with a variably prominent nucleolus [2, 9]. Epithelioid cells are round or polyhedral

Fig. 1. A 57-year-old man presented for decreased vision in the right eye for the past 3 months. Visual acuity was counting fingers in the right eye and 20/20 in the left. External examination revealed a blue iris with absence of melanocytosis or heterochromia. Sentinel vessels were absent. Anterior segment examination of both eyes and dilated fundus examination of the left eye were unremarkable. In the right eye, the medium was clear and the optic disk was normal. Located in the nasal quadrant, a dome-shaped pigmented choroidal tumor with irregular surface was noted (**a**). Ultrasonography revealed basal dimensions of 20 × 15 mm and a height of 9.0 mm (**b**). Low internal reflectivity was present on A scan (**c**). The tumor was classified as large sized (COMS criteria), and enucleation was performed. The enucleation specimen has a ciliochoroidal melanoma with the characteristic dark coloration (**d**). FNAB of the enucleation specimen yielded mostly spindle cells, some with marked nuclear atypia including enlarged nuclei and prominent nucleoli (**e**, Papanicolaou stain). Tissue sections also showed similar marked nuclear atypia (**f**, hematoxylin and eosin stain).

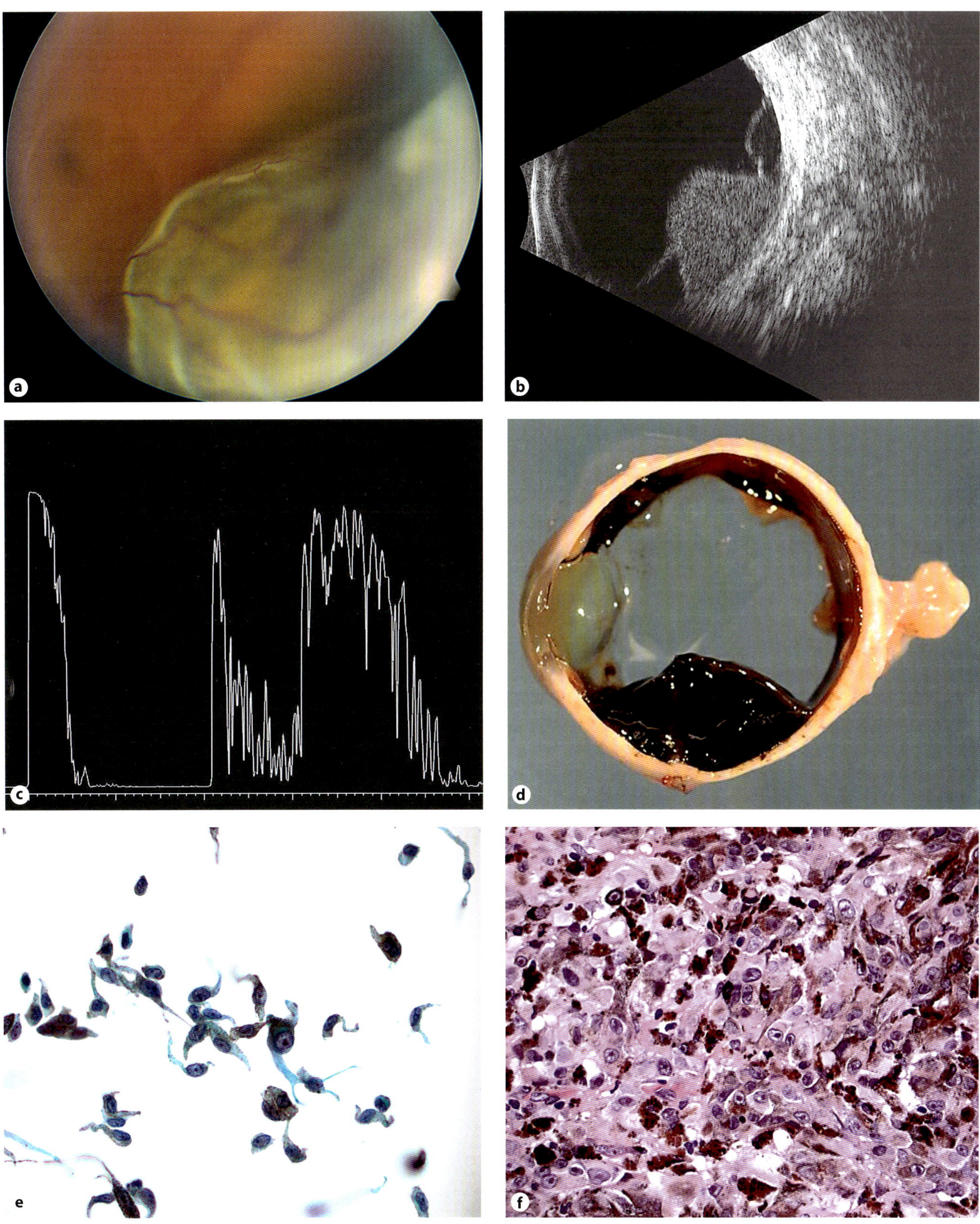
a
b
c
d
e
f

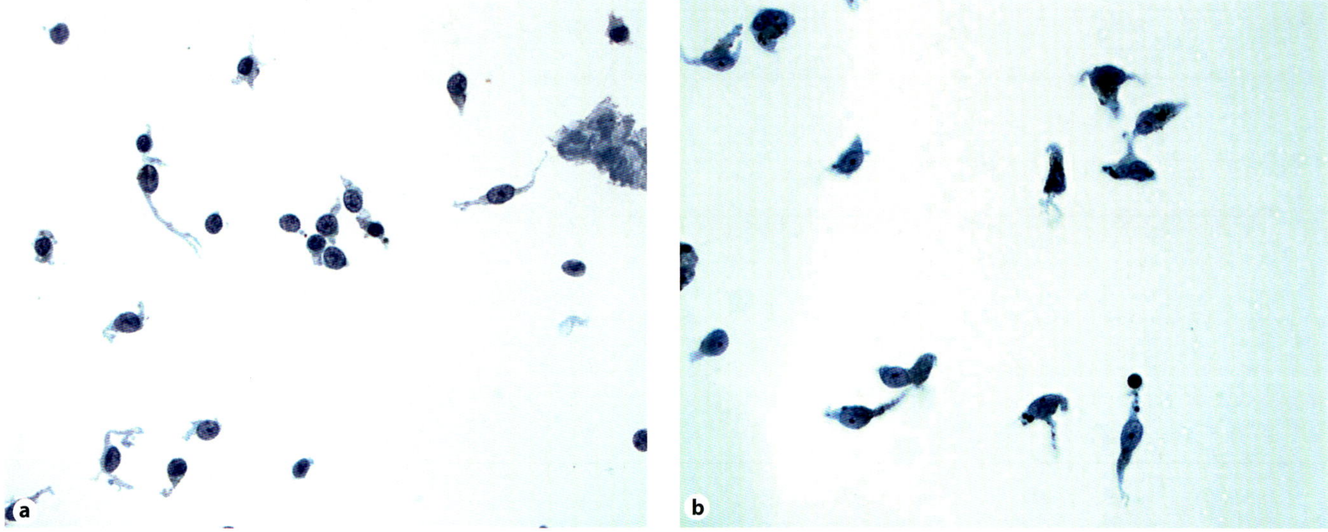

Fig. 2. Uveal melanoma cells typically have relatively bland nuclear features. In this example, spindle cells and rare epithelioid cells have conspicuous nucleoli but relatively uniform nuclear size, shape and chromatin pattern (**a**). This spindle cell melanoma has the typical relatively uniform nuclei with fine chromatin and small but distinct nucleoli. Papanicolaou stains (**b**).

and usually have larger nuclei and more prominent nucleoli [2, 9].

Sample Adequacy

Adequacy is the most important limiting factor for uveal FNAB [10]. The cellular diagnosis of uveal melanoma involves FNAB of solid masses. Exfoliative cytology is ineffective. In particular, vitreous fluid samples are not indicated because uveal melanoma cells rarely involve the vitreous due to the retina's resistance to invasion [8].

Experienced clinicians working closely with cytologists usually obtain adequate samples as illustrated by the 88–95% reported adequacy rates [1, 11]. Cellular yield relates directly to lesion size [12, 13], and adequacy has been more of an issue for small uveal lesions as evidenced by the 65% adequacy rate in a series of uveal melanocytic lesions having a maximal basal diameter of 10 mm and a thickness between 1.5 and 3 mm [13]. A positive uveal FNAB diagnosis is reliable but a negative diagnosis must be interpreted with caution and, with rare exceptions (see the differential diagnosis section), not considered proof of benignancy [14]. In fact, even a negative histopathological diagnosis does not guarantee a benign lesion in many cases [15], in part because of the potential for sampling error and confusion created by the relatively bland cells of spindle cell melanoma [1, 16].

Cytological Features

FNAB samples from uveal melanomas have characteristic cellular features. Surprisingly to most cytopathologists, uveal melanomas typically have a relatively bland cellular appearance (fig. 2) due to the prevalence of spindle cells (fig. 3) and the fact that spindle cell melanomas have bland cellular features [2, 17]. At least some spindle cells are usually present, often associated with an epithelioid component creating a mixed pattern in most cases (fig. 4). In our experience 78% of FNAB samples, from uveal melanoma, had at least a component of spindle cells [18]. Spindle cells have a fusiform or multipolar cytoplasmic shape (fig. 3). Spindle cell nuclei vary from round to oval or elongate and usually have fine orthochromatic chromatin and variable, often inconspicuous nucleoli [2]. In contrast, epithelioid cells have a round or polyhedral shape (fig. 5) [9]. The epithelioid shape associates with classical nuclear features of malignancy, notably nuclear enlargement, pleomorphism and prominent nucleoli [2]. Further, epithelioid cells vary in size and shape often having an abundant amphophilic cytoplasm and a plasmacytoid configuration [2]. Intranuclear cytoplasmic invaginations are typical of the epithelioid cell type and are therefore a helpful differential diagnostic criterion [2]. Cytoplasmic melanin is a consistent feature (fig. 3). We identified it in 78% of cases though only after diligent search in some [18]. Melanin granules are small and finely distributed in contrast to the larger

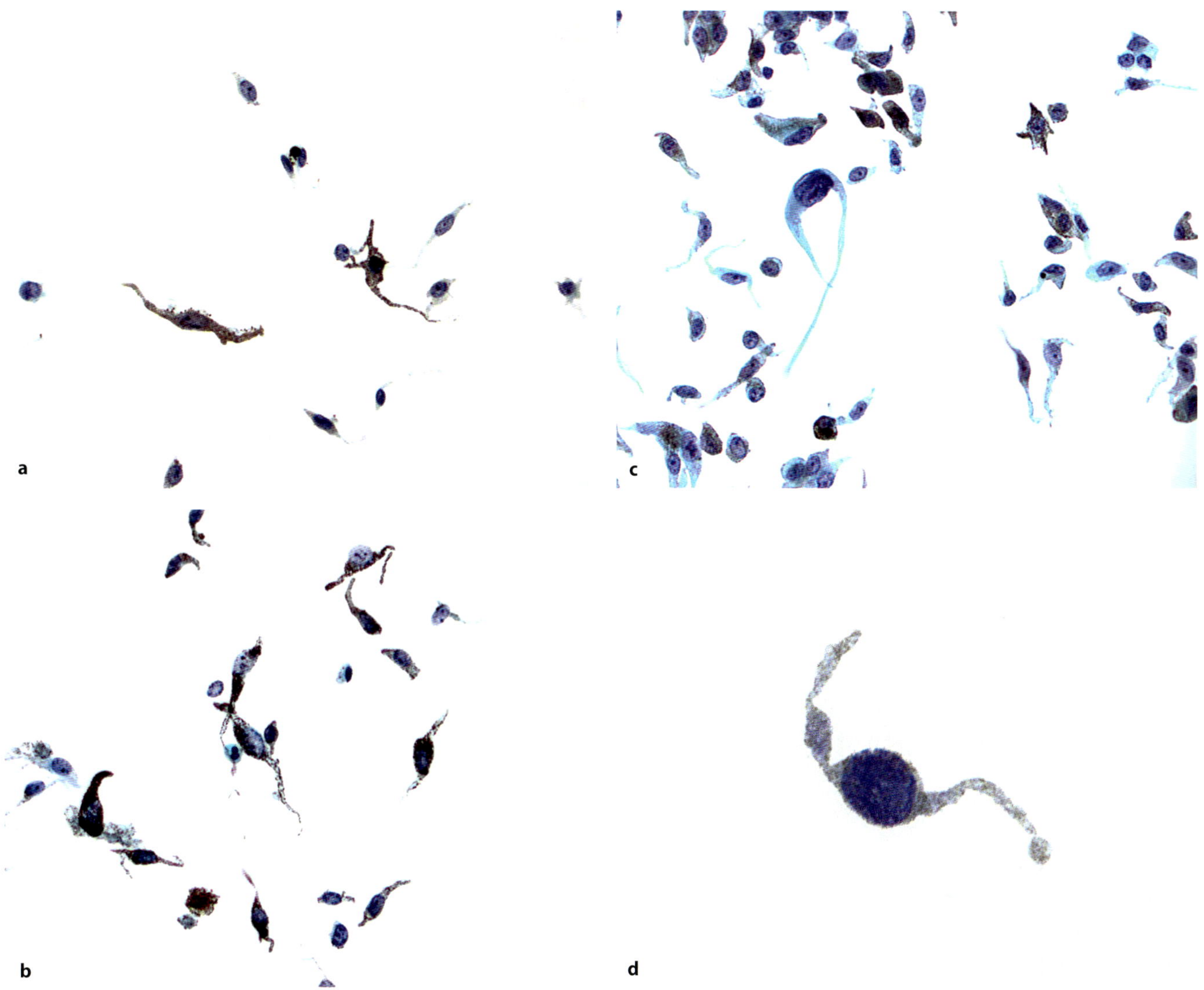

Fig. 3. Spindle cell shape, especially a slender caudate cytoplasm, is a helpful differential diagnostic cytological feature. Note typical bland nuclear features (**a**, **b**), marked nuclear atypia (**c**) and caudate cytoplasm (**d**). Papanicolaou stains.

and coarser phagocytosed hemosiderin and melanin granules and histiocytes.

Special Considerations

Iris Melanoma

Cytologists must be aware of some peculiarities of iris melanocytic lesions. Understandably due to location, iris lesions present earlier in their natural history. As a result, patients are younger and lesions smaller [9, 19]. Importantly, melanocytic iris lesions are predominantly benign. In fact, in an analysis of 103 iris lesions originally histologically diagnosed as melanoma, 75 (73%) were reclassified as benign [9]. Further, no tumor deaths occurred in the approximately 13% of patients assigned to the melanoma group after review. Fifteen-year survival for iris melanoma approximates 95% in contrast to approximately 55% for posterior uveal (choroid and ciliary body) melanomas [5, 9]. In one series, only 1 (4%) patient with histologically confirmed iris melanoma died of disease [5]. Iris melanoma accounts for only 2–5% [2, 5] of uveal melanomas but iris lesions are sampled more often in part due to easier access compared to posterior uveal lesions. Note that only approximately 2.5% of ocular tumors in general undergo diagnostic FNAB [1] while up to 7% of iris tumors are subjected to diagnostic FNAB

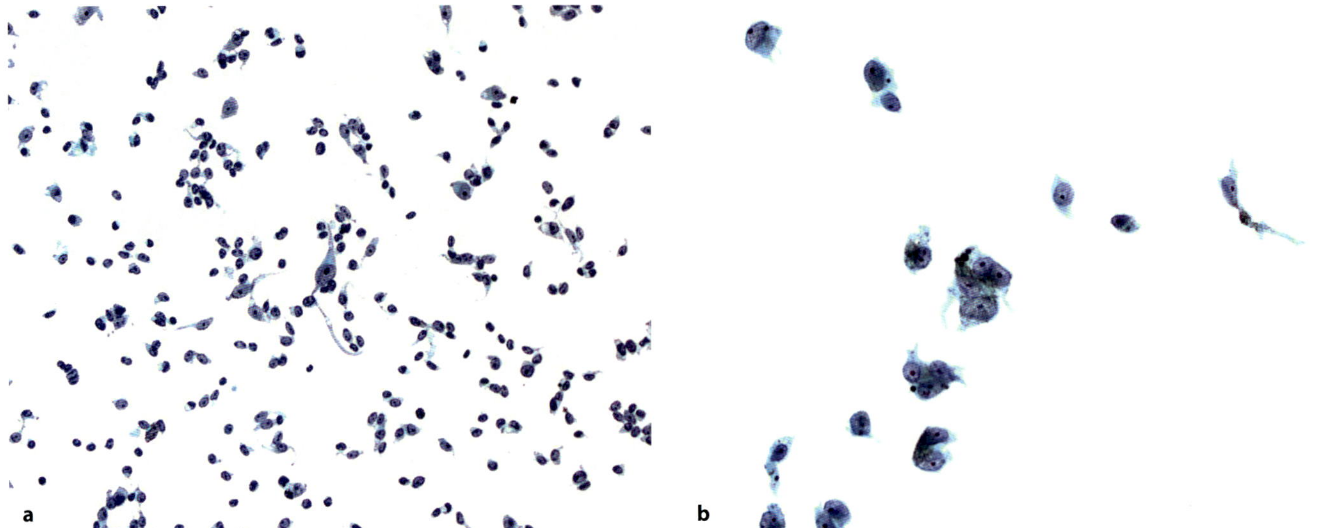

Fig. 4. Uveal melanoma aspirate samples usually have a mixed spindle cell and epithelioid cell pattern as illustrated by these samples from two different tumors (**a**, **b**). Papanicolaou stains.

[4]. Compared to choroidal and ciliary body melanocytic lesions, iris lesions more often have bland spindle cells [9] which must be interpreted within the clinical context and in concert with the ophthalmologist, in order to confirm a diagnosis of melanoma.

Prognostic Features

Morphological variables correlate with the prognosis for uveal melanoma. Established histological prognostic variables include cell type, nucleolar size, necrosis, mitoses, tumor-infiltrating lymphocytes and macrophages, vascular density, extravascular matrix patterns, extent of pigment deposition and scleral invasion [Chapter 6, this vol., pp. 55–60; 2, 8]. Some of these histological features easily translate to cytology including cell type, nucleolar size and tumor-infiltrating lymphocytes. Epithelioid cell type was the first histological feature linked to prognosis [8]. Epithelioid appearance closely associates with other cellular features classically associated with malignant behavior including nuclear enlargement, pleomorphism, necrosis and mitoses (fig. 5). Therefore, the presence of epithelioid cells should be reported by the cytologist [2]. Interestingly, in contrast to their significance in malignancies at other sites, tumor-infiltrating lymphocytes (fig. 6) are associated with an increased risk of metastases in uveal melanoma [8]. In our ongoing study of uveal melanomas aspirated for prognostication, we identified tumor-infiltrating lymphocytes in 23% of cases [unpubl. data].

Not surprisingly, the epithelioid phenotype is associated with epithelial-like molecular changes including expression of cytokeratin, E-cadherin and β-catenin as well as increased gene expression of epithelial adhesion markers [2]. Interestingly expression of E-cadherin and its localization in the plasma membrane rather than the cytoplasm have been associated with aggressive behavior in other tumors including melanoma [2]. These molecular changes have been proposed to explain the association between the epithelioid morphological phenotype and malignant behavior [2]. In contrast, spindle cell melanoma more closely resembles nonneoplastic uveal melanocytes at the morphological and molecular level [2].

Secondary Changes/Artifacts

Various FNAB approaches to uveal lesions can introduce contamination into the aspirate sample. For example, the common pars plana transvitreous approach can rarely introduce conjunctival contamination (fig. 7). Retinal pigment epithelium could also contaminate a transvitreous sample but, in our experience, this must be a vanishingly rare occurrence. Secondary changes can complicate the interpretation of uveal melanoma. Specifically, necrosis and hemorrhage can obscure the cellular detail (fig. 7) [1]. Pigment-laden macrophages can be confused for melanoma cells. Macrophages have lower nuclear-to-cytoplasmic ratios and often eccentric and reniform nuclei [9]. Pigment within macrophages tends to be coarser and more granular.

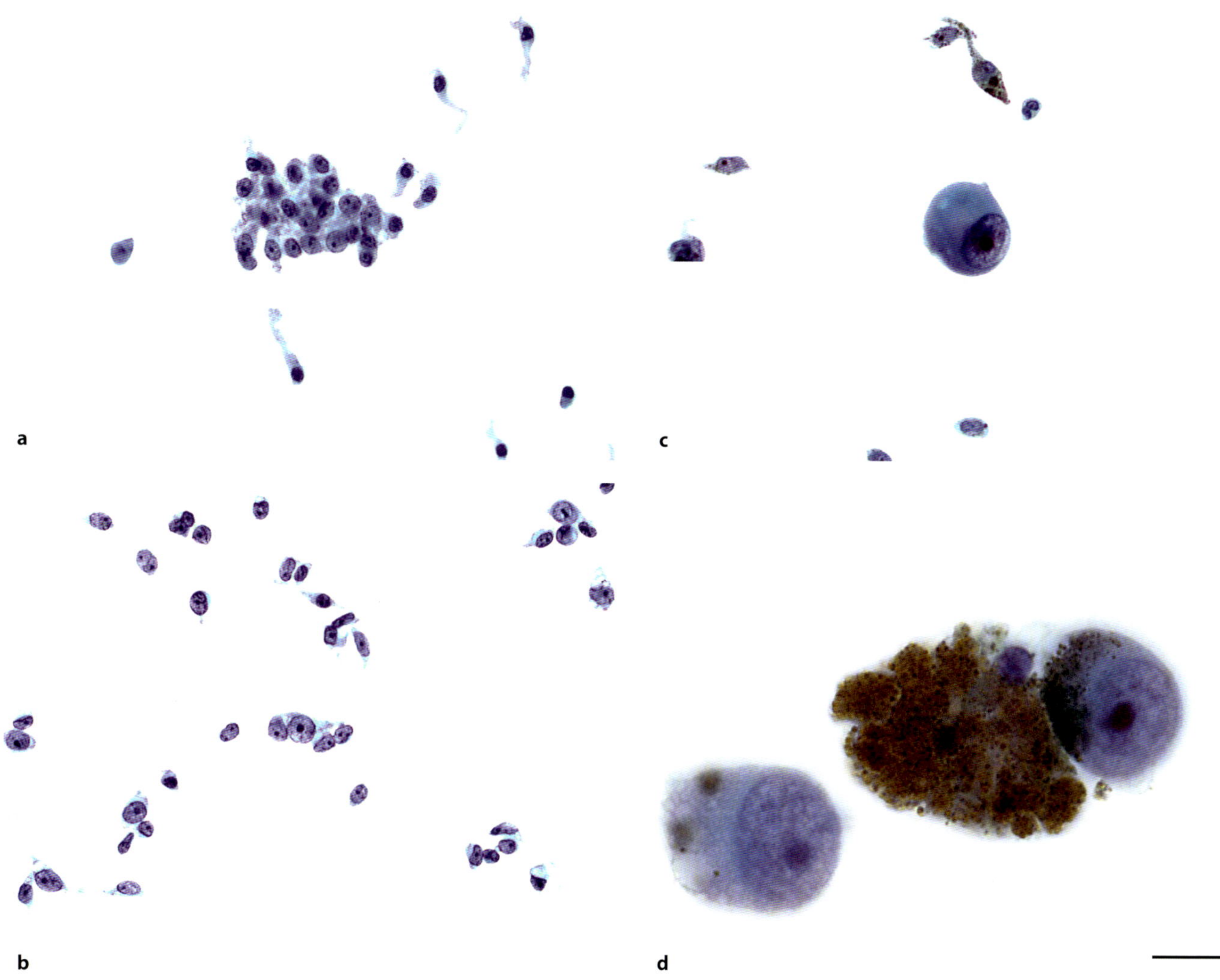

Fig. 5. The epithelioid appearance associates with an increased risk of metastases. Further, uveal melanoma cells with epithelioid shape can be confused with metastatic carcinoma, as illustrated by the aggregate of epithelioid melanoma cells (**a**). The characteristic spindle-shaped cells, also evident in this image, provide a clue to the diagnosis. Nuclear atypia and pleomorphism are more commonly seen with the epithelioid cell type (**b**, **c**). These two epithelioid melanoma cells were imaged with an oil immersion ×100 objective (**d**). Papanicolaou stains. Scale bar = 10 µm. Courtesy of Judy Drazba, PhD.

Clinical Scenarios

Benign Pigmented Proliferations

Importantly, FNAB can effectively diagnose some benign melanocytic uveal lesions. Melanocytoma has sufficiently distinctive cellular features including large, regular pigment granules that obscure or obliterate the nuclear detail and small bland nuclei, apparent after melanin bleach [2, 20]. Interestingly, melanocytoma more commonly affects adults of African or Asian descent in contrast to the marked predilection for uveal melanomas to affect light-skinned individuals [2]. A pigmented epithelial layer lines the inner margin of the retina and extends anteriorly to the ciliary body and the posterior aspect of the iris [2]. In contrast to melanoma, adenomas of this pigmented epithelium have cohesive clusters of uniform epithelial cells with bland nuclear features and, large regular spherical pigment granules in contrast to the fine dusting of melanin pigment

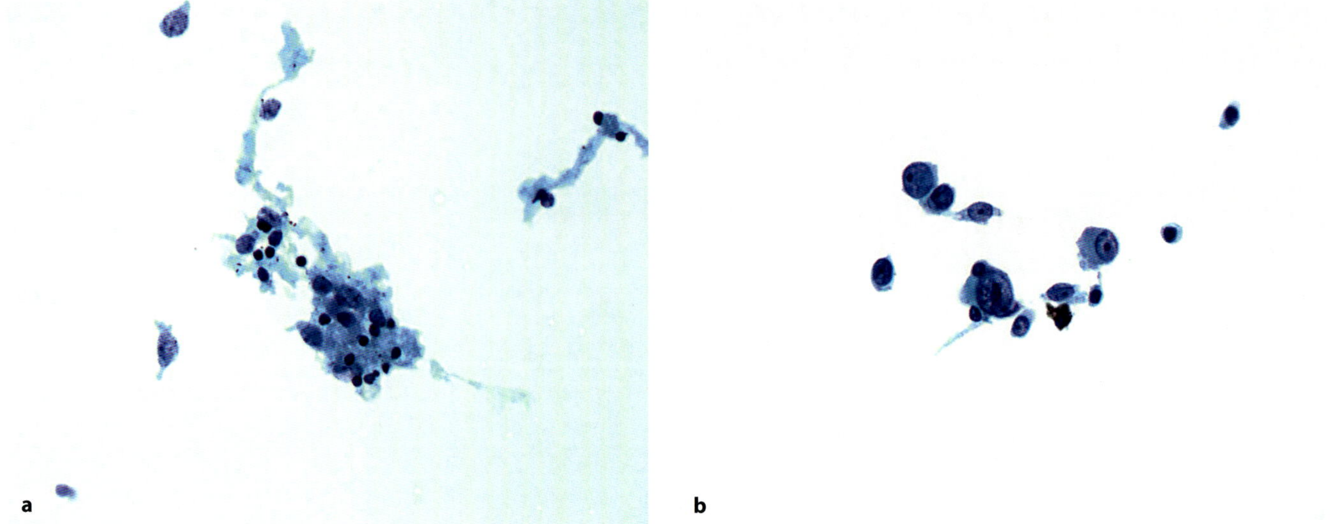

Fig. 6. In tissue sections, tumor-infiltrating lymphocytes are an adverse prognostic variable. They can be recognized in aspirate samples. Lymphocytes infiltrate aggregates of uveal melanoma cells (**a**) and articulate with the cytoplasm of an epithelioid uveal melanoma cell (**b**). Papanicolaou stains.

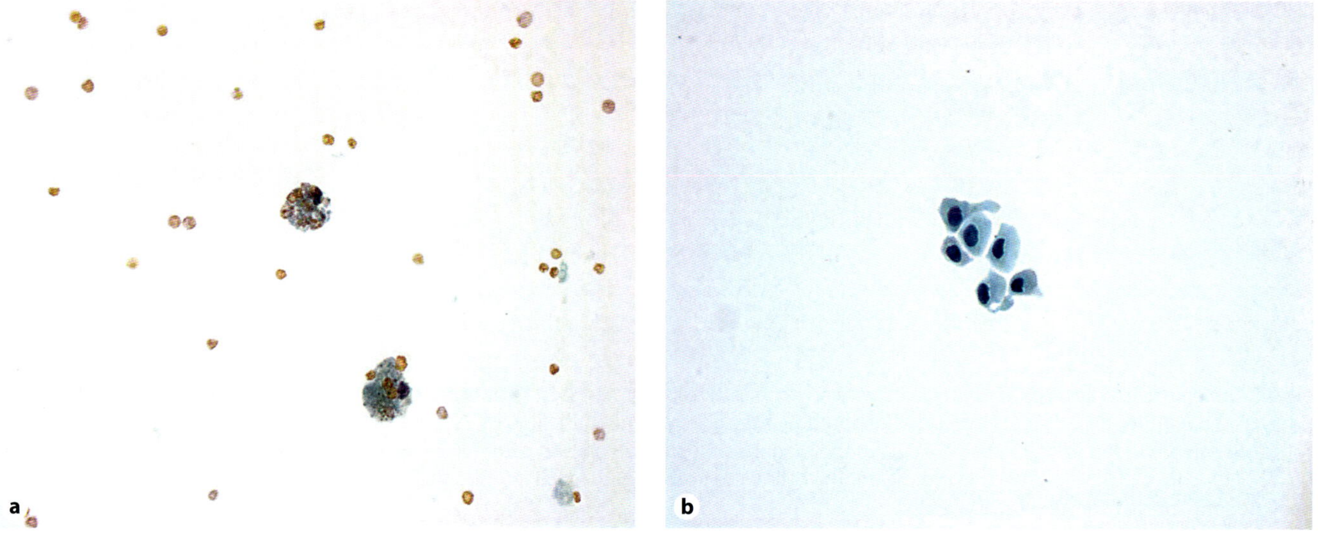

Fig. 7. Hemorrhagic uveal melanoma may contribute to a false-negative FNAB interpretation. In this example, aspirate material contains only red blood cells and histiocytes (**a**). Contaminants acquired along the needle tract can complicate FNAB interpretation. This sample from a pars plana transvitreous approach contains benign epithelial cells interpreted as conjunctival epithelial contamination (**b**). Papanicolaou stains.

characteristic of melanoma [2, 20]. Note that retinal pigment epithelial adenocarcinomas have been reported albeit vanishingly rarely. These are recognized clinically by locally aggressive growth with invasion into adjacent structures [2].

Nevus versus Melanoma (Indeterminate Melanocytic Lesions)

FNAB has utility in the differential diagnosis of uveal nevus versus melanoma but cytologists must understand some important limitations of FNAB in this setting. Firstly, uveal nevi and melanomas are defined, in part, by size. Specifically, regarding choroidal lesions, the collaborative melanoma study group defines choroidal nevus as less than or equal to 5 mm in basal diameter and less than or equal to 1 mm in height [16]. Choroidal lesions greater than 1 mm but less than 2.5 mm in height and greater than 5 mm but less than or equal to 16 mm in basal dimension are regarded as small melanoma but we prefer the designation indeterminate melanocytic lesion because 60% of these lesions remain stable and follow a benign clinical course [16, 21].

FNAB has limitations in the evaluation of these small melanocytic lesions. Firstly, adequacy is more of an issue because cell yield directly relates to lesion size. Witness the fact that in one study of small melanocytic choroidal tumors in the differential diagnosis of nevus versus melanoma, 35% of the FNAB samples were inadequate and another 12% were indeterminate [13]. Further, the decreased cellularity contributes to sampling error which is an important cause of false-negative FNAB [16]. Finally, cytologists struggle to distinguish spindle cell nevus from spindle cell melanoma and spindle cells predominate in uveal melanomas, especially the smaller lesions [2]. Importantly, a positive cytological diagnosis in the differential of nevus versus melanoma is reliable [1, 14]. The presence of conventional cytological criteria of malignancy is diagnostic of melanoma. Specifically, look for the epithelioid cell type. Epithelioid shape alone is not sufficient since epithelioid nevi occur in the iris and the posterior uvea, albeit they are extremely rare [2, 9]. Importantly, epithelioid cells almost always have malignant cellular features including prominent nucleoli and nuclear pleomorphism [2, 22]. Remember that uveal nevi, by definition, have fine orthochromatic chromatin and inconspicuous or absent nucleoli [9, 23].

In summary, in the differential diagnosis of nevus versus melanoma, a positive cellular diagnosis is reliable [1, 13, 14, 22] but a negative diagnosis should be interpreted with caution and not embraced as definitive evidence of a benign lesion [1, 20]. Notably, experienced ophthalmic oncologists have concluded that small melanoma versus large nevus is a relative contraindication to FNAB because of the diagnostic difficulties noted above [1].

Uveal Melanoma and Metastasis

Published experience supports uveal FNAB to confirm malignant diagnoses including melanoma and metastases. Augsburger et al. [14] examined 71 ocular FNA samples. Forty-four of these were performed on surgical specimens, with 41 of those being done on solid tumors. Twenty-seven of the biopsies were performed preoperatively to establish the diagnosis. Of those 27 biopsies, 16 were done to confirm a malignancy and 11 were to confirm a benign diagnosis. Ten of the 16 biopsies done to confirm a malignancy were for melanoma while 4 were for suspected metastases, 1 for suspected retinoblastoma and 1 for suspected medulloepithelioma. Fifteen (93.8%) of these cases were diagnosed as malignant on cytology. Histological correlation was available for 9 of those and the cytological diagnoses were confirmed in 8 out of 9 cases. One of the 9 proved to be false positive. The false-positive case and the one benign case were both melanocytomas. All 11 aspirates done to confirm benign conditions were read as benign [14].

Shields et al. [1] have also reported on the diagnostic effectiveness of intraocular FNA on 140 patients with intraocular malignancies such as uveal melanoma, uveal metastasis, retinoblastoma, lymphoma and leukemia. A histological correlation was available in 57 of cases, with histology-cytology diagnostic concordance in 54 of 57 (95%) cases.

Davila et al. [24] obtained follow-up data on 17 patients diagnosed as either suspicious or positive for malignancy on ocular cytology samples at their institution. Their report included 9 vitreous, 6 anterior chamber and 3 FNA samples. A histological follow-up was available in 6 cases with diagnostic agreement seen in 5 cases (83%). The one discordant case was of fungal endophthalmitis diagnosed as 'suspicious for lymphoma'. Overall, the cytological interpretation matched the follow-up clinical and histological data in 11 of 12 (92%) patients for whom it was available [24].

Eide et al. [25] reported on 80 patients presenting for intraocular FNA with inconclusive intraocular disease. They found FNA to be accurate and helpful in clinical decision-making with adequate material being received in 77 of 80 cases. FNA interpretations precluded enucleations for 25 patients, including 16 with benign lesions. One melanoma was incorrectly interpreted as a metastasis [25].

Stepwise Diagnostic Evaluation

Regardless of the differential diagnosis, cytologists must interpret the cellular features within the clinical context. This emphasizes the importance of communication between cytologists and ophthalmologists.

First Step

Metastasis should be the first differential diagnostic consideration because metastases are the most common uveal malignancy, and approximately two thirds of uveal FNABs are performed to resolve a clinical differential diagnosis that includes metastasis and melanoma [1]. Cytologists should

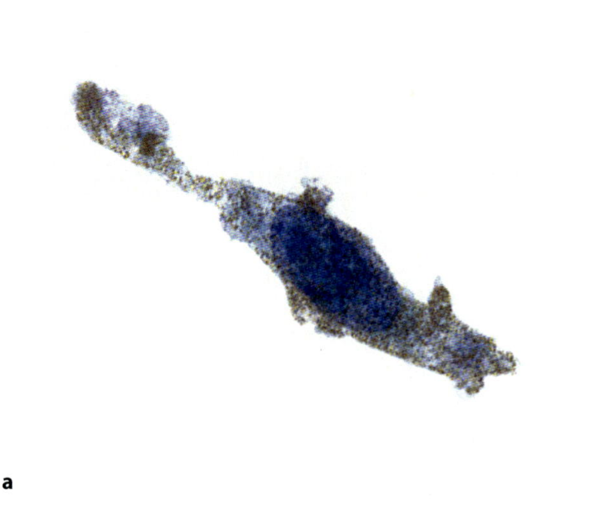

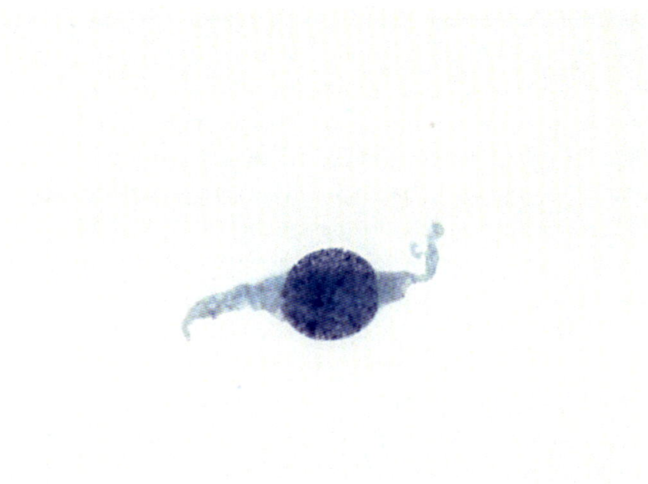

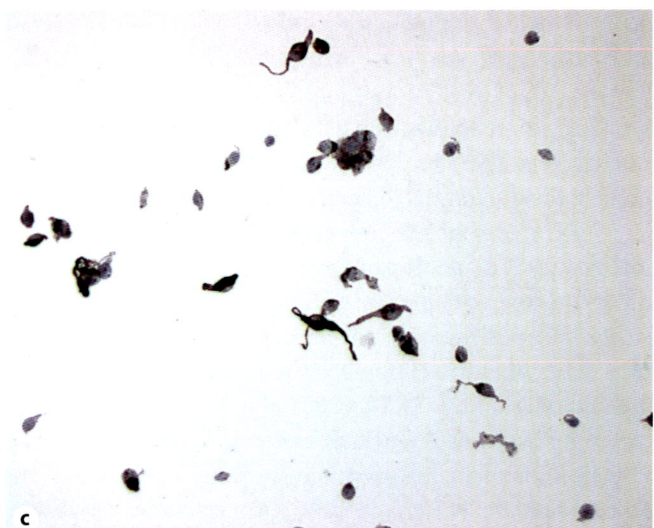

Fig. 8. Presence of melanin and spindle cells is a helpful cytological diagnostic feature. This uveal melanoma cell has melanin and is spindle shaped (**a**). This spindle cell lacks melanin (**b**). Though rarely needed, immunohistochemical stains for melanoma markers, such as HMB45 illustrated here, can help identify amelanotic melanoma cells (**c**).

first look for cytoplasmic melanin pigment (fig. 3, 8). Be aware that melanin can be focal and inconspicuous, especially in samples from clinically ambiguous cases. We found melanin in 78% of uveal melanomas in our small series of aspirates performed for diagnosis [18]. Melanin has a finely granular cytoplasmic distribution.

Second Step

The spindle type melanoma cell (fig. 3, 8) is the next most helpful diagnostic criterion in the differential diagnosis with metastasis because the vast majority of uveal metastases are carcinomas, mostly from the breast and lung (fig. 9) [26]. These tumors have an epithelioid appearance and more cohesive cell clusters. Spindle cell carcinomatous metastases occur rarely and include squamous carcinoma and neuroendocrine carcinomas [27]. In contrast to spindle cell melanoma, squamous metastases have more cohesive aggregates, and the cells have a more densely staining cytoplasm and sharper cytoplasmic borders. The characteristic stippled chromatin pattern helps to recognize neuroendocrine carcinomas. Other spindle cell neoplasms including leiomyoma and sarcoma must also be considered. Leiomyomas generally lack the multipolar dendritic shape of some spindle cell melanoma cells. Sarcomas rarely metastasize to the uvea. When indicated, comparison to a known primary (sarcoma) or immunohistochemistry (leiomyoma) for smooth muscle markers such as actin and desmin can be helpful.

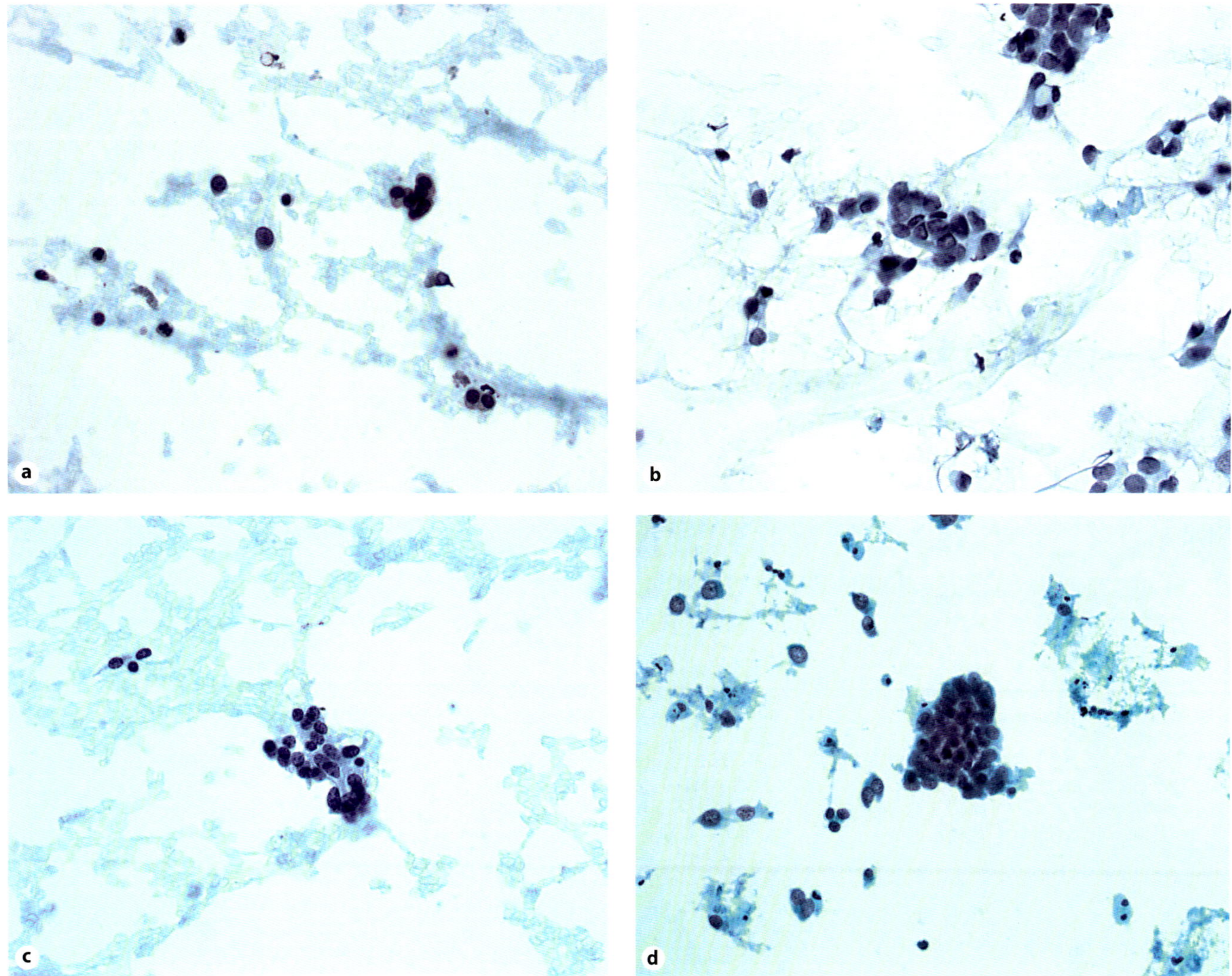

Fig. 9. Breast and lung carcinomas dominate among the sources of metastases to the uvea. Lobular breast carcinoma can be subtle with relatively small adenocarcinoma cells distributed individually and in small aggregates (**a**). Ductal breast carcinoma typically has more overtly malignant nuclear features (**b**). Typical bronchial carcinoid tumor has the relatively bland nuclei with stippled chromatin characteristic of low-grade neuroendocrine carcinomas (**c**). Aggregates and individual carcinoma cells characterize this pulmonary adenocarcinoma (**d**). Papanicolaou stains.

Third Step

Immunohistochemistry for epithelial markers including cytokeratins, neuroendocrine markers and melanoma markers such as S100 and HMB45 can be helpful especially in cases of amelanotic epithelioid cell melanoma (fig. 5) [3]. Faulkner-Jones et al. [3] examined the effectiveness of FNAB on solid intraocular tumor management in 33 patients. Specifically they reported on the effect of immunohistochemistry on the positive predictive value, sensitivity and specificity of cytology. Immunohistochemistry was found to increase the positive predictive value and specificity from 93 to 96% and 67 to 83%, respectively. There was no change observed in the sensitivity. A histological follow-up was available in 12 patients and showed agreement with the cytological interpretation in 10 (83%) cases [3]. While published reports on the use of immunohistochemistry in intraocular FNAB specimens are limited, others have also shown it to be an effective diagnostic tool [25, 28].

However, in our experience immunohistochemistry is rarely needed. Importantly, two thirds of patients with uveal metastases have a known primary malignancy. Review of that lesion and comparison usually obviate the need for immunohistochemistry. We have found immunohistochemistry useful for suggesting primary tumor sites in cases of intraocular metastases with no known primary tumor and in diagnosing melanocytic lesions.

Conclusions

A potential issue for cytologists is the struggle with well-differentiated spindle cell melanoma versus spindle cell nevus. Fortunately in many instances, nevus is not a clinical consideration. Consider the fact that confirmation of a clinical diagnosis of metastasis or confirmation of a clinical diagnosis of melanoma are the two most common indications for uveal FNAB. Thus, a valid question for cytologists to pose is: 'Is nevus a diagnostic consideration?' If not, the cytologist can focus on recognizing melanocytic differentiation versus metastasis. Importantly, cytologists should not be asked to confirm a clinical impression of nevus, since ophthalmoscopic appearance combined with small size and stable growth are reliable clinical criteria.

References

1 Shields JA, Shields CL, Ehya H, Eagle RC Jr, De Potter P: Fine-needle aspiration biopsy of suspected intraocular tumors: the 1992 Urwick lecture. Ophthalmology 1993;100:1677–1684.
2 Ylagan LR: Intraocular pigmented proliferations in the context of cytologic evaluation. Diagn Cytopathol 2009;37:853–864.
3 Faulkner-Jones BE, Foster WJ, Harbour JW, Smith ME, Davila RM: Fine needle aspiration biopsy with adjunct immunohistochemistry in intraocular tumor management. Acta Cytol 2005;49:297–308.
4 Shields CL, Manquez ME, Ehya H, Mashayekhi A, Danzig CJ, Shields JA: Fine-needle aspiration biopsy of iris tumors in 100 consecutive cases: technique and complications. Ophthalmology 2006;113:2080–2086.
5 Char DH, Crawford JB, Kroll S: Iris melanomas: diagnostic problems. Ophthalmology 1996;103: 251–255.
6 Shields JA, Shields CL, De Potter P, Singh AD: Diagnosis and treatment of uveal melanoma. Semin Oncol 1996;23:763–767.
7 Callender G: Malignant melanocytic tumors of the eye: a study of histologic types in 111 cases. Trans Am Acad Ophthalmol Otolaryngol 1931; 36:131–142.
8 Kivela T: Uveal malignant melanoma: histopathologic features; in Singh AD, Damato BE, Pe'er J, Murphree AL, Perry JD (eds): Essentials of Ophthalmic Oncology. Thorofare, Slack, 2009, pp 219–225.
9 Jakobiec FA, Silbert G. Are most iris 'melanomas' really nevi? A clinicopathologic study of 189 lesions. Arch Ophthalmol 1981;99:2117–2132.
10 Char DH, Kemlitz AE, Miller T, Crawford JB: Iris ring melanoma: fine needle biopsy. Br J Ophthalmol 2006;90:420–422.
11 Char DH, Miller T: Accuracy of presumed uveal melanoma diagnosis before alternative therapy. Br J Ophthalmol 1995;79:692–696.
12 Cohen VM, Dinakaran S, Parsons MA, Rennie IG: Transvitreal fine needle aspiration biopsy: the influence of intraocular lesion size on diagnostic biopsy result. Eye (Lond) 2001;15:143–147.
13 Augsburger JJ, Correa ZM, Schneider S, et al: Diagnostic transvitreal fine-needle aspiration biopsy of small melanocytic choroidal tumors in nevus versus melanoma category. Trans Am Ophthalmol Soc 2002;100:225–232.
14 Augsburger JJ, Shields JA, Folberg R, Lang W, O'Hara BJ, Claricci JD: Fine needle aspiration biopsy in the diagnosis of intraocular cancer: cytologic-histologic correlations. Ophthalmology 1985;92:39–49.
15 Schalenbourg A, Uffer S, Zografos L: Utility of a biopsy in suspicious pigmented iris tumors. Ophthalmic Res 2008;40:267–272.
16 Singh AD: Tumors of the uvea: benign melanocytic tumors; in Singh AD, Damato BE, Pe'er J, Murphree AL, Perry JD (eds): Essentials of Ophthalmic Oncology. Thorofare, Slack, 2009, pp 185–197.
17 Kashyap S, Sen S, Sharma MC, Sethi A: Diagnostic intraocular aspiration cytology of choroidal melanoma. Diagn Cytopathol 2002;26:389–391.
18 Baker SE, Fu E, Weber D, Biscotti CV: The role of fine needle aspiration in the evaluation of uveal tumors: a clinicopathologic analysis of 26 consecutive cases. Can Cytopathol 2008;114:357–358.
19 Geisse LJ, Robertson DM: Iris melanomas. Am J Ophthalmol 1985;99:638–648.
20 Char DH, Miller TR, Crawford JB: Cytopathologic diagnosis of benign lesions simulating choroidal melanomas. Am J Ophthalmol 1991;112:70–75.
21 Collaborative Ocular Melanoma Study Group: Factors predictive of growth and treatment of small choroidal melanoma: COMS report No 5. Arch Ophthalmol 1997;115:1537–1544.
22 Char DH, Miller TR, Ljung BM, Howes EL Jr, Stoloff A: Fine needle aspiration biopsy in uveal melanoma. Acta Cytol 1989;33:599–605.
23 Folberg R: Uveal malignant melanoma: prognostic factors, in Singh AD, Damato BE, Pe'er J, Murphree AL, Perry JD (eds): Essentials of Ophthalmic Oncology. Thorofare, Slack, 2009, pp 272–276.
24 Davila RM, Miranda MC, Smith ME: Role of cytopathology in the diagnosis of ocular malignancies. Acta Cytol 1998;42:362–366.
25 Eide N, Syrdalen P, Walaas L, Hagmar B: Fine needle aspiration biopsy in selecting treatment for inconclusive intraocular disease. Acta Ophthalmol Scand 1999;77:448–452.
26 Shields CL, Shields JA, Gross NE, Schwartz GP, Lally SE: Survey of 520 eyes with uveal metastases. Ophthalmology 1997;104:1265–1276.
27 Trichopoulos N, Augsburger JJ: Neuroendocrine tumours metastatic to the uvea: diagnosis by fine needle aspiration biopsy. Graefes Arch Clin Exp Ophthalmol 2006;244:524–528.
28 Pelayes DE, Zarate JO: Fine needle aspiration biopsy with liquid-based cytology and adjunct immunohistochemistry in intraocular melanocytic tumors. Eur J Ophthalmol 2010;20:1059–1065.

Charles V. Biscotti, MD
Department of Anatomic Pathology, Cleveland Clinic Foundation
9500 Euclid Avenue
Cleveland, OH 44195 (USA)
Tel. +1 216 444 0046, E-Mail biscotc@ccf.org

Chapter 6

Biscotti CV, Singh AD (eds): FNA Cytology of Ophthalmic Tumors.
Monogr Clin Cytol. Basel, Karger 2012, vol 21, pp 55–60

Uveal Melanoma: Prognostication

Mary E. Turell[a] · Raymond R. Tubbs[b] · Charles V. Biscotti[c] · Arun D. Singh[a]

[a]Cole Eye Institute, [b]Molecular Genetic Pathology and [c]Department of Anatomic Pathology, Cleveland Clinic Foundation, Cleveland, Ohio, USA

Despite successful treatment of the primary tumor, uveal melanoma carries a significant risk of developing metastatic disease, which occurs almost uniformly in the liver. The cumulative melanoma-related mortality 25 years following treatment is approximately 52% for individuals with medium-sized tumors [1]. Most experts agree that micrometastases exist at the time of ophthalmic diagnosis, and perhaps even precede clinically recognizable ophthalmic disease [2]. Micrometastases may remain dormant for prolonged intervals before manifesting as macrometastatic disease [3]. Unfortunately, once uveal melanoma has spread to distant organs, the disease is largely resistant to currently available therapies [4].

Recently, significant progress has been made in understanding the role of tumor histopathology, cytogenetics and gene expression patterns in predicting metastatic potential. For this reason, it has become increasingly common to perform tissue biopsy by means of fine needle aspiration (FNA) for prognostic purposes. Fluorescence in situ hybridization (FISH), single-nucleotide polymorphism (SNP) array and gene expression profiling (GEP) are frequently employed to assess metastatic risk. Indications for FNA and surgical technique are discussed elsewhere [Chapter 1, this vol., pp. 1–9].

Prognostic Factors

Cytological Features

In addition to confirming the diagnosis of uveal melanoma, FNA is useful for assessing several cytological indicators of prognosis. Cell type was the first feature to be correlated with survival [5, 6]. In general, uveal melanomas composed of epithelioid cells (fig. 1) are considered to be more aggressive than their spindle cell or mixed cell counterparts (fig. 2). Challenges in interobserver variation, for example lack of consensus as to the number of epithelioid cells required to distinguish mixed from epithelioid cytology, are problematic. An increased number of mitotic figures has consistently been demonstrated to correlate with poorer prognosis [7]. Other cytological features such as high numbers of tumor-infiltrating lymphocytes are also associated with adverse outcomes (fig. 3) [7–10].

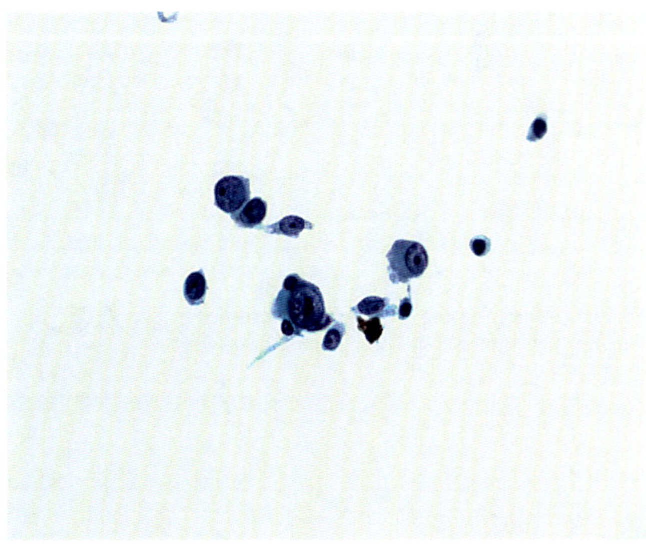

Fig. 1. Epithelioid melanoma cells have a round or polyhedral shape. They also often have more overtly malignant nuclear features including enlargement and prominent nucleoli. These cells were derived from a uveal melanoma. Papanicolaou stain.

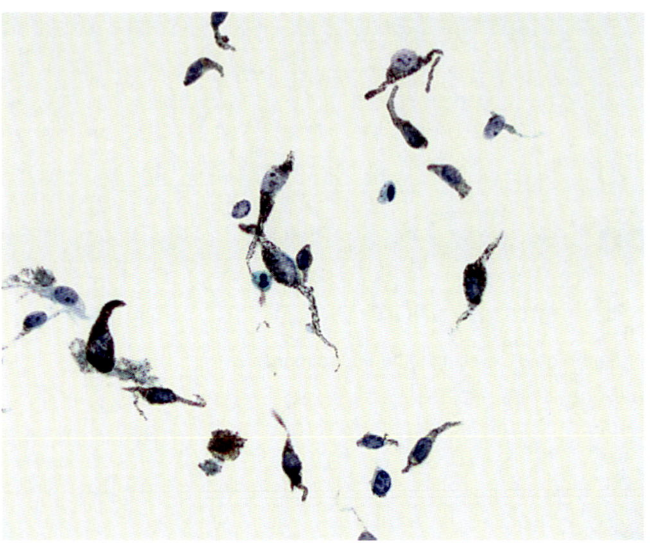

Fig. 2. Spindle melanoma cells have a fusiform shape, often with dendritic cytoplasm. These cells were derived from a prominently pigmented uveal melanoma. Papanicolaou stain.

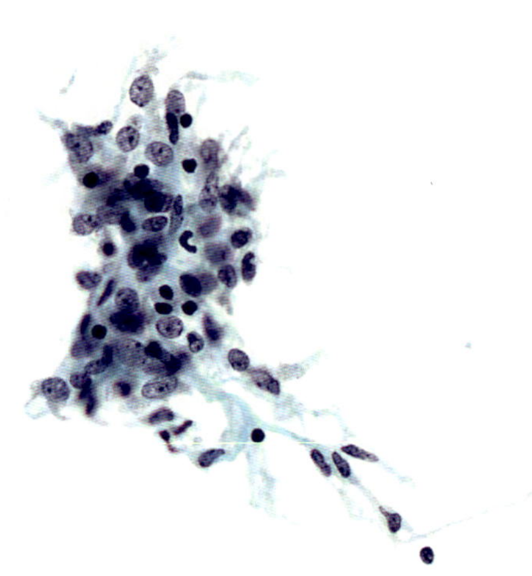

Fig. 3. Lymphocytes infiltrate a cluster of uveal melanoma cells. Papanicolaou stain.

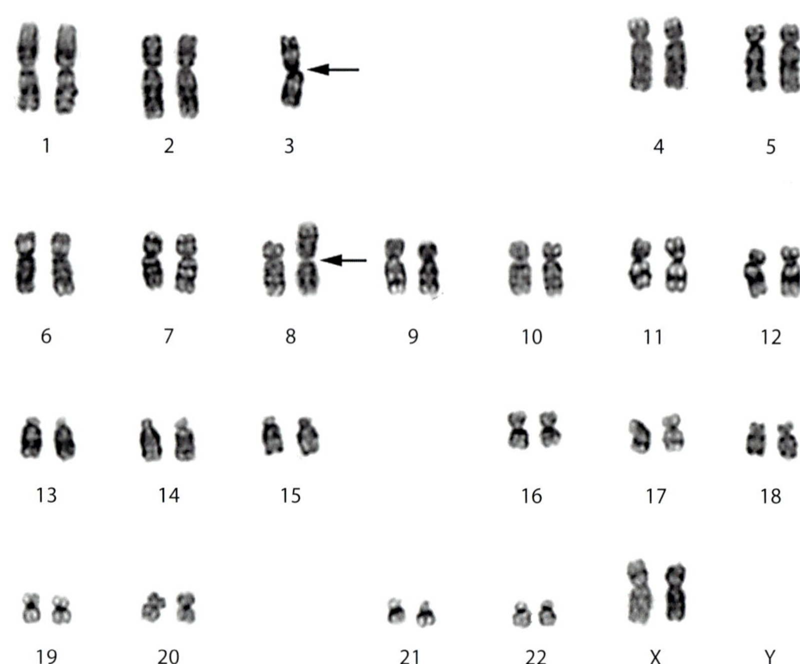

Fig. 4. Karyotype of a uveal melanoma showing loss of chromosome 3 and isochromosome 8q (arrows). Reproduced with permission from Singh et al. [15].

Standard Karyotyping

Uveal melanoma cytogenetic research began in the early 1990s with standard karyotyping [11–13]. Tumor cells that exhibited minimal chromosomal aberrations were found to be similar to early cutaneous melanomas and were not associated with an increased risk of mortality when followed for extended periods [14]. The first reported genetic abnormalities in uveal melanoma were found to involve chromosomes 1, 3, 6 and 8 (fig. 4) [12, 13]. In 1992, Horsthemke et al. [11] and Prescher et al. [16] proposed that aberrations

macrophages or retinal pigment epithelial cells in tissue biopsies (fig. 3) [19].

In the presence of a granulomatous inflammation and negative staining for fungi, mycobacteria and other microorganisms, the diagnosis of sarcoidosis (fig. 3), Behçet disease (fig. 3) or granulomatosis with polyangiitis should be considered, if the history and clinical findings are consistent with this condition. In younger patients, juvenile xanthogranulomatosis characterized by the Touton giant cells, should be considered, particularly in anterior uveal lesions. Exceptionally rarely, intranuclear and intracytoplasmic viral inclusion bodies (e.g. cytomegalovirus or herpes simplex virus) may be demonstrated in association with necrotic cells in the vitreous or chorioretinal samples. Such inclusion bodies are, however, usually seen in chorioretinal biopsies, using immunohistochemical or immunofluorescence techniques (fig. 3). PCR analysis of ocular fluid samples may expedite the diagnosis and early treatment of such conditions, since the retinitis can progress rapidly.

Syphilis, once the main cause of vitreous opacities [1], now accounts for only about 1% of all vitreous opacities but is increasing in incidence, particularly in HIV-positive populations. Essentially, it should always be considered in the differential diagnosis of an inflammatory cellular vitreous infiltrate, particularly with dominance of plasma cells, and can be highlighted in silver stains.

Neoplastic Disease

Malignant neoplasms including primary ocular tumors such as VRL and retinoblastoma, as well as systemic diseases such as leukemia, metastatic carcinomas and metastatic cutaneous melanomas can be diagnosed using vitreous biopsies (fig. 4) [20]. The main neoplastic 'masquerader' to be diagnosed in a vitrectomy specimen is VRL, which is located most often within the subretinal space, with perivascular infiltrates in the retina and seeding into the vitreous [20, 21].

Cytomorphological examination of vitreous infiltrates in VRL demonstrates medium-to-large cells with minimal cytoplasm, large pleomorphic or round (sometimes bare) nuclei and prominent nucleoli (fig. 5). Necrotic material and macrophages are commonly present in the background, causing difficulties in cytological interpretation (fig. 5).

Immunocytology discloses the B-cell nature of the majority of these tumors with expression of CD79a, CD20 and PAX-5 (fig. 5). Many viable neoplastic cells stain positively with the MIB-1 antibody, indicating a high growth fraction, i.e. the high-grade nature of this malignancy. The diagnosis of lymphoma is supported by demonstration of cellular monotypical expression of either a light and/or heavy chain of the immunoglobulin gene (usually IgM) [22, 23]. Should sufficient material be available for examination, investigation of the vitreous specimens for rearrangements of the immunoglobulin heavy chain gene using PCR provides further evidence for the diagnosis of VRL (fig. 6).

Biochemical analysis of the vitreous specimen for interleukin ratios (IL-10:IL-6) may also support the diagnosis of VRL [24]. If possible, VRL should be distinguished from other types of intraocular lymphoma, namely primary uveal lymphoma (fig. 5) and secondary ('metastatic') intraocular lymphomas, which are usually of non-Hodgkin type [20]. In such cases, the clinical history and examination findings are particularly important in bringing all aspects together in an integrated report.

Nondiagnostic Vitreous Biopsy

A 'negative' tumor biopsy is particularly problematic and disappointing for all involved in cases of intraocular malignancy as: (a) it fails to provide a diagnosis in a case of a suspected neoplasm and (b) fails to provide prognostication information to patients whose demands for such information are increasing. The causes of failed intraocular biopsies are many. First of all, the bioptic material may not contain any material of diagnostic relevance, for example, vitreous in primary uveal lymphomas, and in some cases of VRL where the tumor cells are 'hidden' in the subretinal space with minimal vitreal involvement. Secondly, the patient may

Fig. 3. Vitreous biopsy comprised mainly of macrophages but with occasional scattered toxoplasmosis cysts (arrow) (**a**, Periodic acid-Schiff. ×40). Vitreous biopsy of an immunosuppressed patient with a dense infiltrate of macrophages containing numerous Ziehl-Neelsen-positive bacilli within their cytoplasm (**b**, Ziehl-Neelsen. ×60). Chorioretinal biopsy with a noncaseating granulomatous reaction in a patient with uveitis and vitreitis, due to *Histoplasma capsulatum* (**c**, Periodic acid-Schiff. ×60). Chorioretinal biopsy with a noncaseating granuloma with a Schaumann body (arrow), typical of sarcoidosis (**d**, Hematoxylin-eosin. ×40). Chorioretinal biopsy of a young patient with extensive anterior and posterior uveitis, retinitis and uveitis, due to Behçet disease: a typical granuloma with multinucleate cells and scattered eosinophils (**e**, arrow). Vitreous biopsy containing dense fibrovascular membranes with plump endothelial cells and scattered cells (**f**), with clear intranuclear inclusion bodies of cytomegalovirus (**g**, alkaline phosphatase/anti-alkaline-phosphatase complex, ×40), and chorioretinal biopsy (**h**, hematoxylin-eosin, ×40) in a patient with retinal necrosis, vasculitis and vitreitis, caused by herpes simplex (**inset**).

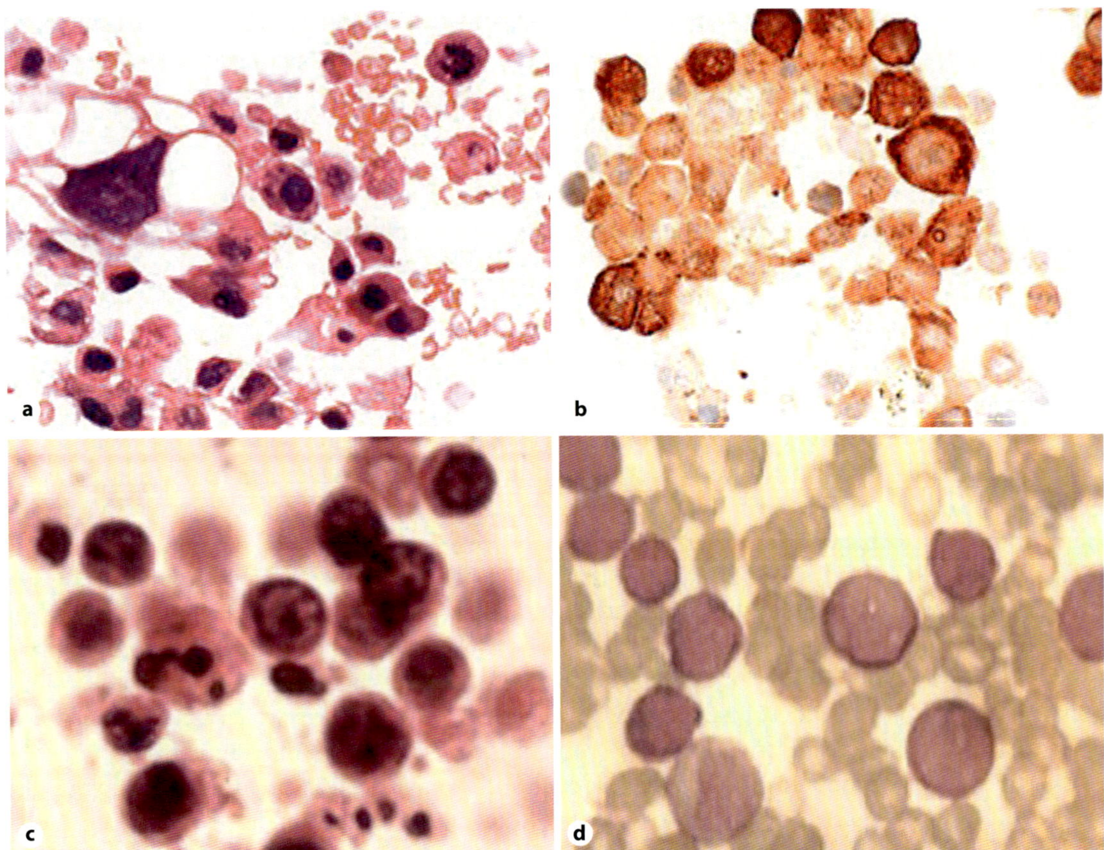

Fig. 4. Vitreous biopsy with scattered atypical cells with moderate eosinophilic cytoplasm and large pleomorphic and anaplastic nuclei, in a patient with metastatic cutaneous melanoma (**a**, Hematoxylin-eosin. ×40). Immunoreactivity of the metastatic cutaneous melanoma cells for Melan A. They were negative for pancytokeratins (**b**, Alkaline phosphatase/anti-alkaline-phosphatase complex. ×40). Vitreous tap of an unsuspected retinoblastoma in a 25-year-old patient, demonstrating small- to medium-sized cells with minimal cytoplasm and dense chromatin within the nuclei. Note scattered apoptotic bodies (**c**, Hematoxylin-eosin. ×40). Hemorrhagic vitreous biopsy with scattered large cells, pale granular cytoplasm and nuclei, characteristic of a myeloid origin (**d**, Hematoxylin-eosin. ×40).

have been treated with medications (e.g. steroids) prior to intraocular biopsy (e.g. vitrectomy), increasing tumor cell fragility. Thirdly, the size of the biopsy sample may be insufficient, for example, containing only scanty tumor cells on a background of hemorrhage. It is therefore recommended that an undiluted vitreous sample of about 1 ml be collected prior to starting the infusion during vitrectomy [25]. Fourthly, the specimen may not be handled properly, for example, not being placed in the correct fixative or being left unfixed for an excessive time. Fifthly, the specimen may have been lost on the way to the laboratory or during laboratory processing (e.g. a tiny retinal biopsy), perhaps as a result of a technical error. Most of these problems can be avoided by taking the precautions already mentioned in this article, and by working closely with an experienced biomedical scientist and reporting pathologist. Whenever a nondiagnostic biopsy occurs, it is especially important for the clinician and pathologist to confer without delay so that any similar errors can be avoided if the investigation is repeated.

Conclusions

The diagnostic workup of vitreous biopsies demands close collaboration between the clinician, the pathologist and the microbiologist. Documentation of all relevant clinical information in the pathology request form as well as timely discussions between the various specialists (for example, telephone communications just before a vitreous biopsy is performed) are essential components of the diagnostic

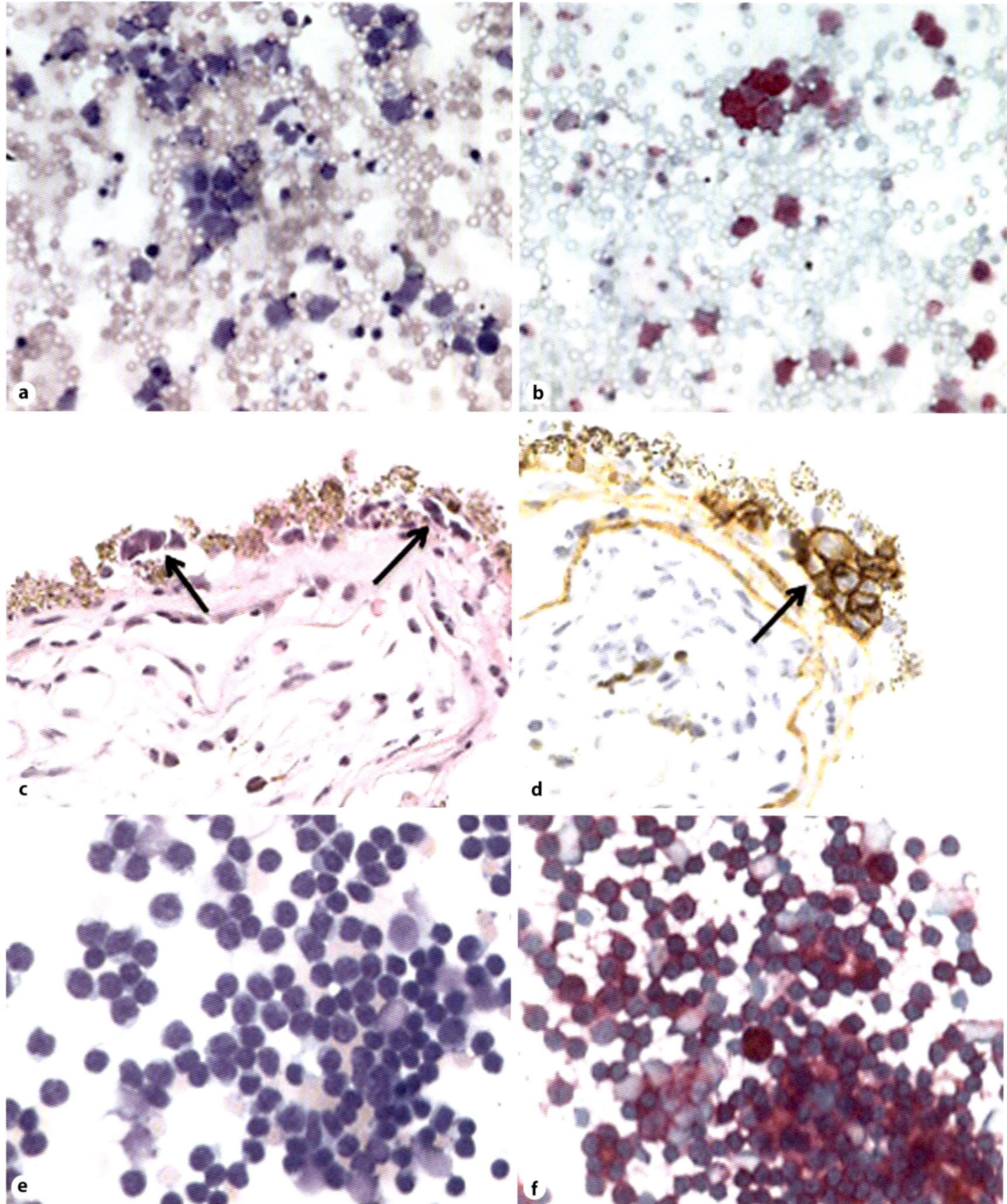

Fig. 5. Hemorrhagic vitreous specimen with scattered large atypical cells with varying amounts of cytoplasm, pleomorphic nuclei and prominent nuclei, characteristic of a VRL (**a**, May-Grünwald-Giemsa. ×20). Immunoreactivity of the neoplastic B cells for the B-cell antigen PAX-5 (**b**, Alkaline phosphatase/anti-alkaline-phosphatase complex. ×20). Chorioretinal biopsy was required to make the diagnosis of VRL in this case, where the neoplastic lymphocytes were confined to the subretinal space (arrows) (**c**, Hematoxylin-eosin. ×40). Immunoreactivity of the B cells for another B-cell antigen, CD20 (arrow) (**d**, Papanicolaou. ×40). Choroidal aspirate of a large choroidal mass, which had unusually infiltrated the retina and disseminated into the vitreous. The mass was composed of small centrocyte-like B cells, with very occasional blasts (**e**). These tumor cells were immunoreactive with the B-cell antigen CD20, and were consistent with a primary extranodal marginal zone B-cell lymphoma of the choroid (**f**, Alkaline phosphatase/anti-alkaline-phosphatase complex. ×40).

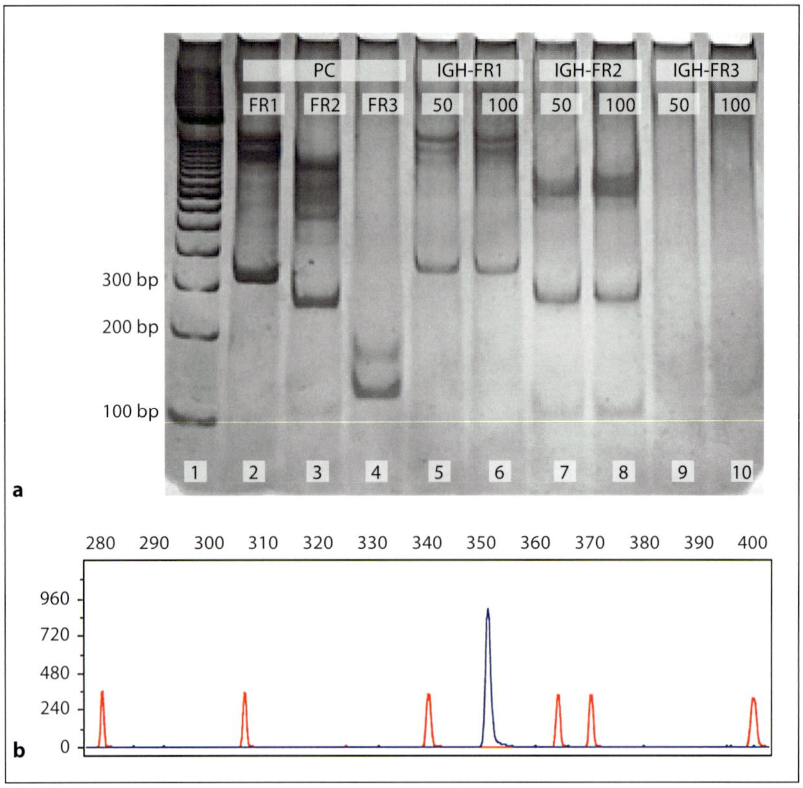

Fig. 6. Image of silver-stained polyacrylamide electrophoresis gel for IgH gene primer sets in a case of VRL. The IgH-PCR was performed on DNA extracted from a vitreous biopsy. Biomed primers are directed against the framework regions 1, 2 and 3 (FR1, FR2 and FR3) of the immunoglobulin heavy chain molecule. The test ladder is on the left of the gel column 1, followed by 3 columns with control samples. The test samples are in differing dilutions in columns 5–10. Monoclonal products were seen using primers FR1 and FR2 in the expected ranges for B-cell amplicates (**a**). Gene Scan sequencing revealed the B-cell clone to be 336 bp in size (**b**, blue peak; red small peaks represent controls). Together with the morphological and immunocytological data, there was sufficient evidence to make an unequivocal diagnosis of VRL in this patient.

pathway, *prior to* specimen arrival in the diagnostic laboratory. The laboratory itself should be equipped with experienced technical staff familiar with the specimen protocols, a pathologist with expertise in ocular pathology/fluid samples, and also be supported with a wide range of investigations, including molecular diagnostic techniques. In this way, the yield from these small samples can be optimized to reach an unequivocal diagnosis, rapid communication to the clinician and timely instigation of therapy.

Acknowledgements

The author would like to thank Prof. B. Damato (Lead of the Liverpool Ocular Oncology Center), Prof. H. Heimann and Mr. C. Groenwald (Consultant Ophthalmologists at the Royal Liverpool University Hospital) as well as vitreoretinal surgeons from Germany, Switzerland and Austria (amongst others, Prof. K.U. Bartz-Schmidt, Prof. N. Bornfeld, Prof. T. Eckhardt, Prof. K. Lemmen, Prof. T. Ness, Prof. M. Zierhut, Prof. M.H. Foerster, Prof. M. Becker and Prof. N. Bechrakis) for the provision of intraocular biopsies for examination. All of the photographs have been included for publication with patient consent.

References

1 Duke-Elder S: Diseases of the vitreous body. System of Ophthalmology. London, Kimpton, 1969.
2 Coupland SE: The pathologist's perspective on vitreous opacities. Eye (Lond) 2008;22:1318–1329.
3 Eide N, Walaas L: Fine-needle aspiration biopsy and other biopsies in suspected intraocular malignant disease: a review. Acta Ophthalmol 2009;87:588–601.
4 Raparia K, Chang CC, Chevez-Barrios P: Intraocular lymphoma: diagnostic approach and immunophenotypic findings in vitrectomy specimens. Arch Pathol Lab Med 2009;133:1233–1237.
5 Coupland SE, Perez-Canto A, Hummel M, Stein H, Heimann H: Assessment of HOPE fixation in vitrectomy specimens in patients with chronic bilateral uveitis (masquerade syndrome). Graefes Arch Clin Exp Ophthalmol 2005;243:847–852.
6 Wang HH, Sovie S, Trawinski G, et al: Thinprep processing of endoscopic brushing specimens. Am J Clin Pathol 1996;105:163–167.
7 Green WR: Diagnostic cytopathology of ocular fluid specimens. Ophthalmology 1984;91:726–749.
8 Mandell D, Levy J, Rosenthal D: Preparation and cytologic evaluation of intraocular fluids. Acta Cytol 1987;31:150–158.
9 Augsburger JJ: Invasive diagnostic techniques for uveitis and simulating conditions. Trans Am Ophthalmol Soc 1990;88:89–104, discussion 104–107.
10 Davis JL, Solomon D, Nussenblatt RB, Palestine AG, Chan CC: Immunocytochemical staining of vitreous cells: indications, techniques, and results. Ophthalmology 1992;99:250–256.

11 Obata H, Horiuchi H, Tsuru T: Clinical application of new membrane filter for cytopathological diagnosis in ophthalmology. Jpn J Ophthalmol1993;37:344–351.
12 Coupland SE, Bechrakis NE, Anastassiou G, et al: Evaluation of vitrectomy specimens and chorioretinal biopsies in the diagnosis of primary intraocular lymphoma in patients with masquerade syndrome. Graefes Arch Clin Exp Ophthalmol 2003;241:860–870.
13 Streeten B: Vitreous asteroid bodies: ultrastructural characteristics and composition. Arch Ophthalmol 1982;100:969–975.
14 Sandgren O, Holmgren G, Lundgren E: Vitreous amyloidosis associated with homozygosity for the transthyretin methionine-30 gene. Arch Ophthalmol 1990;108:1584–1586.
15 Adra CN, Eggerding FA: Diagnostic molecular microbiology in posterior uveitis: principles and applications. Int Ophthalmol Clin 1995;35:75–92.
16 Palkovacs EM, Correa Z, Augsburger JJ, Eagle RC Jr: Acquired toxoplasmic retinitis in an immunosuppressed patient: diagnosis by transvitreal fine-needle aspiration biopsy. Graefes Arch Clin Exp Ophthalmol 2008;246:1495–1497.
17 Font R, Rao N, Issarescu S, McEntee W: Ocular involvement in Whipple's disease: light and electronic microscopic observations. Arch Ophthalmol 1978;96:1431–1436.
18 Fardeau C, Romand S, Rao NA, et al: Diagnosis of toxoplasmic retinochoroiditis with atypical clinical features. Am J Ophthalmol 2002;134:196–203.
19 Rao NA, Saraswathy S, Smith RE: Tuberculous uveitis: distribution of *Mycobacterium tuberculosis* in the retinal pigment epithelium. Arch Ophthalmol 2006;124:1777–1779.
20 Coupland SE, Damato B: Understanding intraocular lymphomas. Clin Experiment Ophthalmol 2008;36:564–578.
21 Mochizuki M, Singh AD: Epidemiology and clinical features of intraocular lymphoma. Ocul Immunol Inflamm 2009;17:69–72.
22 Coupland SE, Heimann H, Bechrakis NE: Primary intraocular lymphoma: a review of the clinical, histopathological and molecular biological features. Graefes Arch Clin Exp Ophthalmol 2004;242:901–913.
23 Chan CC, Wallace DJ: Intraocular lymphoma: update on diagnosis and management. Cancer Control 2004;11:285–295.
24 Merle-Beral H, Davi F, Cassoux N, et al: Biological diagnosis of primary intraocular lymphoma. Br J Haematol 2004;124:469–473.
25 Singh A, Lewis H, Schachat A, Peereboom D: Lymphoma of the retina and CNS; in Singh A, Damato B, Pe'er J, Murphree A, Perry J (eds): Clinical Ophthalmic Oncology. Philadelphia, Saunders-Elsevier, 2007, pp 372–377.

Prof. Sarah Coupland, MBBS, PhD, MRCPath, Consultant Pathologist
Lead Ophthalmic Pathologist and Haematopathologist, Pathology, University of Liverpool
5th Floor Duncan Building, Daulby Street
Liverpool L69 3GA (UK)
Tel. +44 151 706 5885, E-Mail s.e.coupland@liverpool.ac.uk

Biscotti CV, Singh AD (eds): FNA Cytology of Ophthalmic Tumors.
Monogr Clin Cytol. Basel, Karger 2012, vol 21, pp 72–81

Fine Needle Aspiration Biopsy of Retinal Tumors

Mohammad Javed Ali[a] · Santosh G. Honavar[a] · Geeta K. Vemuganti[a] · Arun D. Singh[b]

[a]L.V. Prasad Eye Institute, Hyderabad, India; [b]Cole Eye Institute, Cleveland Clinic Foundation, Cleveland, Ohio, USA

Although there is enough literature on fine needle aspiration biopsy (FNAB) of uveal tumors, the same is not true for retinal tumors, possibly because of the paucity of clear indications and guidelines. Certain general indications and contraindications for FNAB have been formulated based on a review of the literature of published studies [1, 2]. We have listed those that are relevant to retinal tumors (table 1). It has to be emphasized that FNAB is recommended only in highly selected cases where there is a true diagnostic dilemma after all possible clinical investigations including an opinion by an expert ocular oncologist have been obtained. In this chapter, we review such specific indications that may warrant FNAB of frequently encountered retinal tumors.

Retinoblastoma

Retinoblastoma is the most common intraocular malignancy of childhood [3]. The diagnosis is usually made by its typical clinical features using indirect ophthalmoscopy aided by ultrasonography, computed tomography and magnetic resonance imaging as appropriate. Clinical situations that may cause diagnostic confusion in retinoblastoma includes media opacity that precludes tumor visualization, noncalcific tumor, unusual clinical presentation and inappropriate age (>5 years).

FNAB in cases of retinoblastoma or suspected retinoblastoma is generally considered to be a relative contraindication because the risk of seeding of the tumor outside the eye is of particular concern [1, 2, 4]. Retinoblastoma is less cohesive due to large areas of necrosis within the tumor [5]. The current understanding is that owing to the poorly cohesive nature of the tumor, there is a significant possibility of dissemination of neoplastic cells through the needle track [3, 6]. Henkes and Manschot [7] reported a case of retinoblastoma in which extraocular tumor extension occurred 4 months after a transcleral needle biopsy of intraocular tumor. Makley [8] also reported several cases of extraocular extension following intraocular biopsy other than the fine needle aspiration technique. Karcioglu et al. [9] investigated the occurrence of tumor cell seeding in needle tracks following 25-gauge FNAB. The biopsies were done immediately after enucleation, and the needle tracks from the pars plana region were serially sectioned for a detailed histological examination. Clusters of tumor cells were seen in 6 of the 11 needle tracks lending support to the hypothetical risk of tumor seeding and dissemination. Such tumor seeding has also been shown in animal experiments and in in vitro human studies [10, 11]. However, there are a few reports which documented FNAB for retinoblastoma that have not led to extraocular extension [5, 12–14].

The only possible indication for FNAB is in a highly exceptional situation of extreme diagnostic dilemma (fig. 1) [1, 15]. If retinoblastoma is a consideration, the FNAB should be done by a modified technique, wherein the needle is passed parallel to the visual axis through the peripheral cornea, anterior chamber, peripheral iris, zonules (avoiding the lens) and into the suspicious area [1]. Such a technique allows ocular buffer zones and completely bypasses the conjunctiva minimizing the risk of extraocular tumor spread should the condition prove to be a retinoblastoma [1].

Table 1. FNAB of retinal tumors: indications and contraindications

Indications	Major diagnostic uncertainty when there is discrepancy between clinical and noninvasive tests or discrepancy among the noninvasive tests
	Leukocoria in a child but retinoblastoma is not a strong possibility
	An amelanotic fundus lesion in an immunosuppressed patient with diagnostic dilemma to differentiate neoplasm from opportunistic infections
Contraindications	When the diagnosis is reasonably certain based on clinical and noninvasive diagnostic studies
	Diagnostic dilemma where retinoblastoma is a strong suspicion
	The procedure entails major morbidity or worsening of the outcomes

Apart from the dreaded complication of tumor seeding, other possible complications include vitreous hemorrhage that precludes future tumor assessment [1, 2]. The cytological features reported include clusters of small round tumor cells with necrosis and streaming of deoxyribonucleic acid [16]. The extent of differentiation of the retinoblastoma may be variable [17]. Rosettes have been reported but they are rarely identified intact on FNAB [18]. Ultrastructural cytological features of a single case of retinoma (retinocytoma) have also been reported [19].

Lesions Simulating Retinoblastoma

Coats' Disease

A unilateral condition characterized by congenital retinal telangiectasia and exudative retinal detachment in young males, usually presents as leukocoria. Although it has specific features, some rare and atypical cases can be confused with retinoblastoma [20, 21]. FNAB is indicated in such cases. In a large series of FNAB for intraocular tumors, Coats' disease accounted for 4% (5/140) of the cases [1]. Cytopathology usually shows hypocellular smears. Macrophages with a glossy surface are covered and embedded in thick exudates. Cytoplasmic vacuoles, which are presumed to be engulfed lipid, displace the nucleus. Lipid-laden macrophages containing melanin pigment thus support the diagnosis of Coats' disease (fig. 2) [22].

Ocular Toxocariasis

Toxocariasis results from infestation by *Toxocara canis.* It can simulate retinoblastoma by either causing a white fundus granuloma [23] or a diffuse endophthalmitis [24]. FNAB is indicated in atypical cases with diagnostic difficulties. The usual cytology findings include presence of inflammatory cells, predominantly eosinophils. In cases where intraocular infection is a diagnostic possibility, it is important to submit a small portion of the aspirated material for microbiological examination to identify the causative organism (fig. 3) [23]. In addition, evidence of intraocular production of a specific antibody in an aqueous humor sample can assist in establishing the final diagnosis of ocular toxocariasis [25].

Endogenous Endophthalmitis

Endophthalmitis can be confused with retinoblastoma. In two large series of lesions simulating retinoblastoma, 1% of pseudoretinoblastomas was due to infectious causes [26, 27]. Shields et al. [28] have reported 6 cases of endogenous endophthalmitis simulating retinoblastoma. Three of these cases underwent FNAB, and the organisms responsible were *Streptococcus sanguis,* cytomegalovirus and *Candida albicans,* respectively. They recommended that if the eye has potentially useful vision, clinical evaluation suggests endophthalmitis and retinoblastoma is less likely, then FNAB could be performed by the corneal approach. Cytological diagnosis is based on the findings of numerous mature neutrophils and fibrin in the FNAB specimen and the evident microorganisms (fig. 4).

Juvenile Xanthogranuloma

Juvenile xanthogranuloma is an idiopathic inflammatory disorder of young children. Most cases are confined to the skin, but involvement of the iris and posterior uvea is common. The clinical presentation can range from a distinct nodular lesion in the uvea to diffuse iris and chorioretinal infiltration. Spontaneous hyphema is a well-recognized ocular complication. A child with spontaneous hyphema should be evaluated for juvenile xanthogranuloma, retinoblastoma and leukemia [29]. Fine needle aspiration cytology is indicated when the diagnosis is uncertain. Cytopathology demonstrates foamy histiocytes with chronic inflammatory cells and sometimes a typical Touton giant cell (fig. 5).

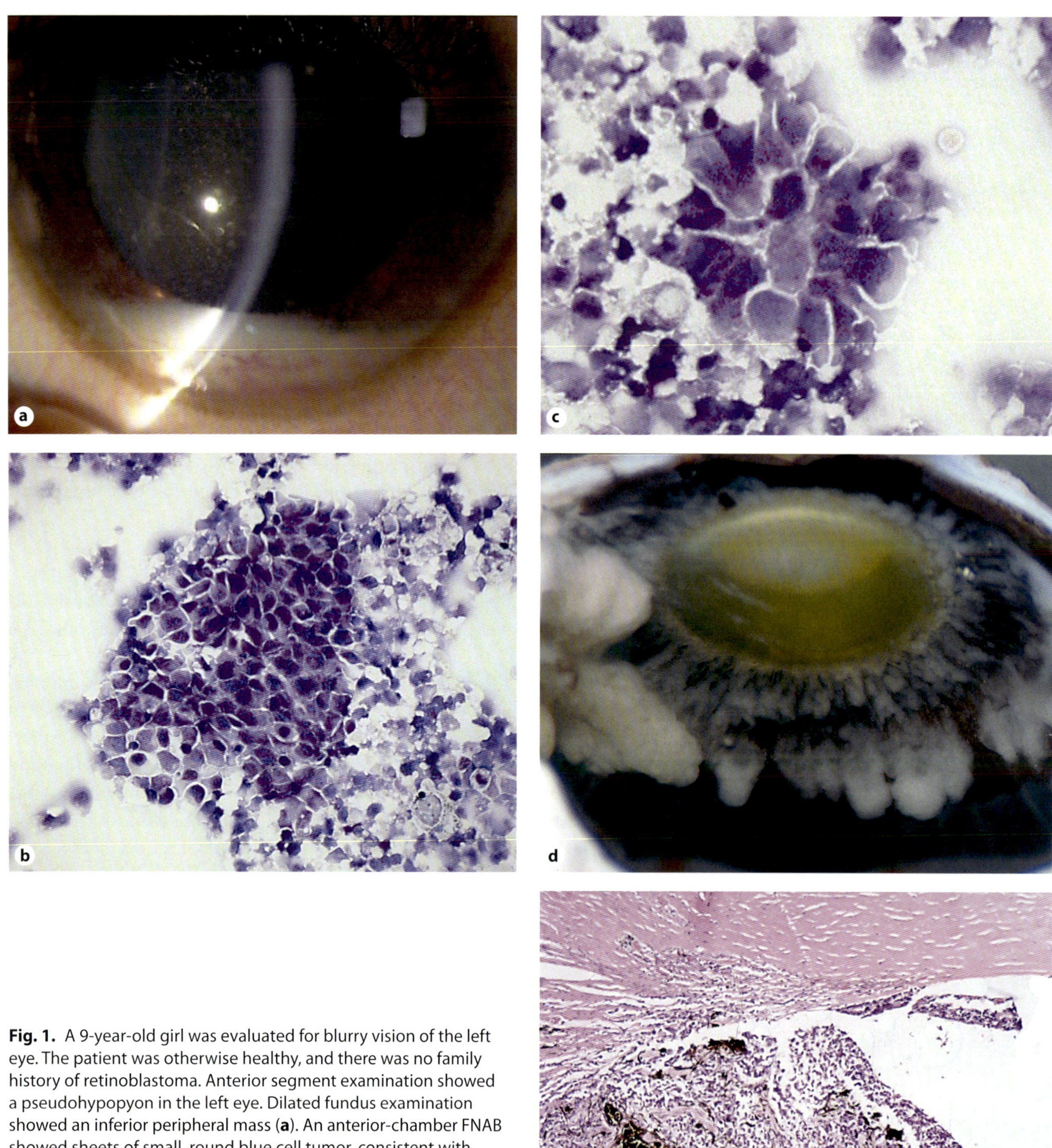

Fig. 1. A 9-year-old girl was evaluated for blurry vision of the left eye. The patient was otherwise healthy, and there was no family history of retinoblastoma. Anterior segment examination showed a pseudohypopyon in the left eye. Dilated fundus examination showed an inferior peripheral mass (**a**). An anterior-chamber FNAB showed sheets of small, round blue cell tumor, consistent with retinoblastoma (**b**). Some of these cells form rosettes (**c**, Wright-Giemsa. Original magnification ×100). Gross anatomical pathology of the enucleated eye revealed 360-degree tumor seeding of the vitreous base and ciliary body (**d**). The tumor cells were present in the anterior chamber, trabecular meshwork, on the iris surface and within the iris (**e**). Reproduced with permission from Crosby et al. [15].

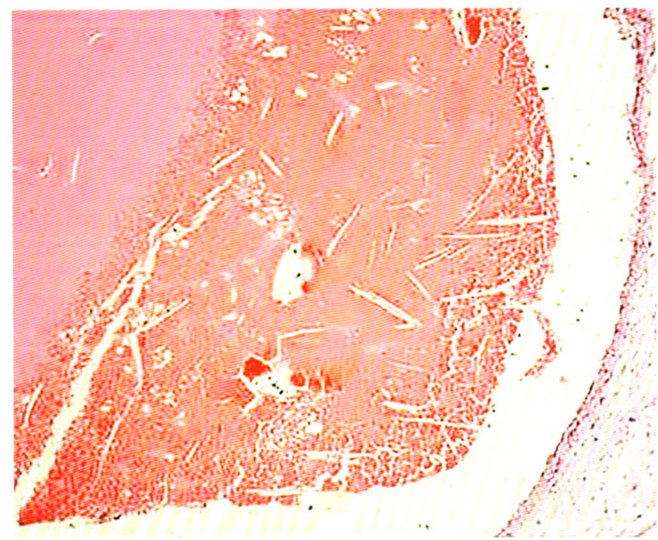

Fig. 2. Coats' disease. Note the anterior segment cholesterolosis. Microphotograph showing numerous lipid-laden crystals. Hematoxylin-eosin. ×100.

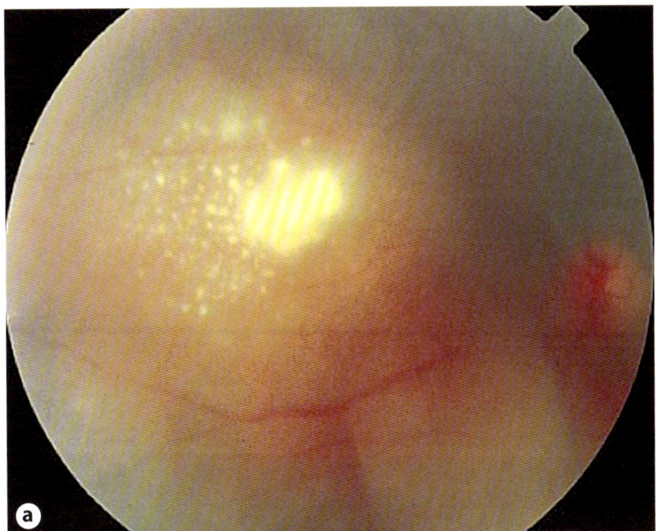

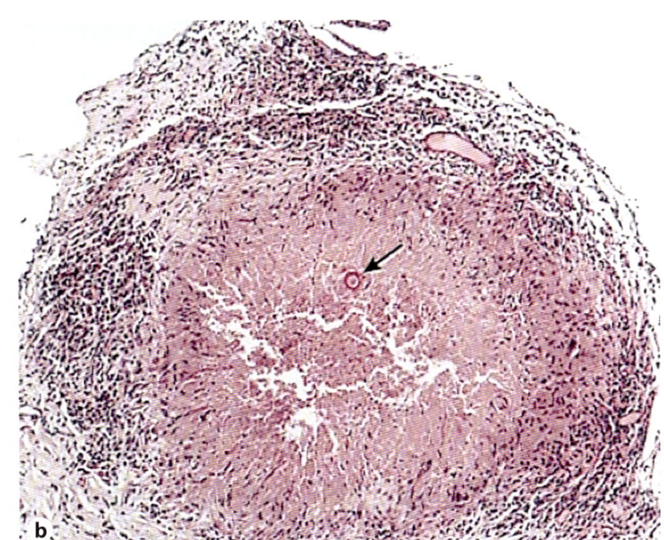

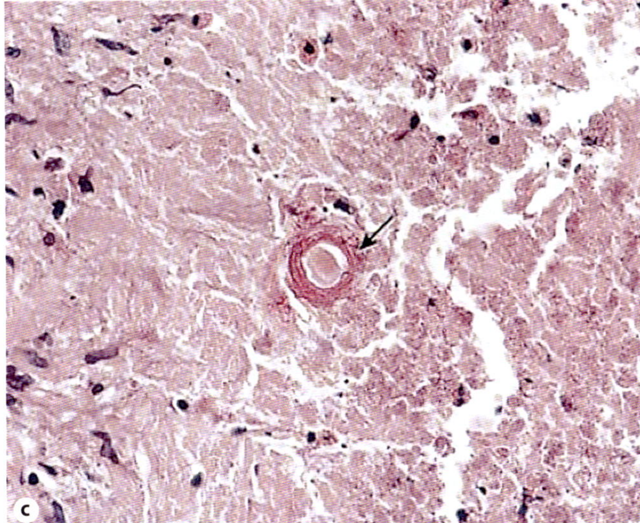

Fig. 3. A 12-year-old boy was evaluated for floaters and decreased visual acuity in his left eye (**a**). Despite treatment for presumed toxoplasmosis, he developed a subretinal mass with vitreous inflammation and macular traction requiring pars plana vitrectomy, membrane stripping, retinotomy, and removal of the epiretinal, retinal and subretinal granuloma. Histological examination identified a necrotic granuloma with a rim of chronic inflammatory cells including lymphocytes, plasma cells and eosinophils. The necrotic zone contains an eosinophilic structure (arrow; **b**, hematoxylin-eosin, original magnification ×188). The central area of necrosis contained an encapsulated eosinophilic structure consistent with a degenerated *Toxocara* larva with the surrounding Splendore-Hoeppli material (arrow; **c**, hematoxylin-eosin, original magnification ×752). Reproduced with permission from Werner et al. [23].

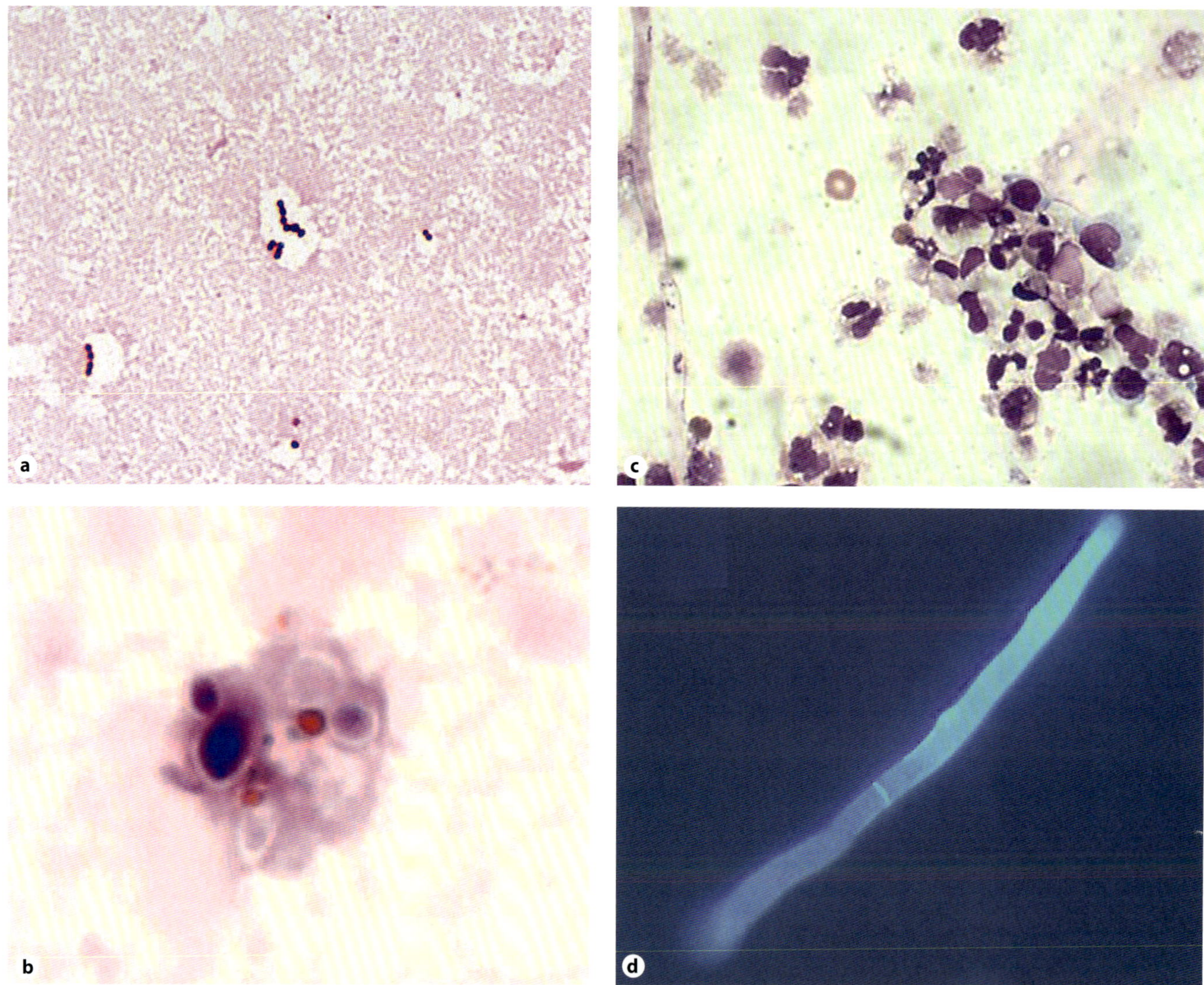

Fig. 4. Cytospin preparations of vitreous fluid show numerous Gram-positive cocci (**a**, Gram stain, ×1,000), budding yeast (**b**, periodic acid-Schiff, ×1,000), septate and branched fungal hyphae (**c**, Giemsa, ×1,000, and **d**, KOH +calcofluor, ×400).

Immunohistochemical staining with CD68 confirms their histiocytic lineage and an S100-negative result helps to differentiate it from other histiocytoses [30].

Medulloepithelioma

Medulloepithelioma is one of the most common nonhereditary embryonal tumors of the nonpigmented ciliary epithelium [31]. Confusion with retinoblastoma can arise in a few atypical cases which present with spontaneous hyphema in a child or when areas of cartilage within the lesion produce echoes similar to dystrophic calcification on ultrasonography [31, 32]. FNAB is rarely indicated in diagnostic dilemmas where retinoblastoma is not a strong suspicion. The usual cytology findings include the presence of cords of benign-appearing small tumor cells. Rosettes are rarely seen (fig. 6).

Retinal Pigment Epithelial Tumors

Retinal pigment epithelium (RPE) tumors may sometimes simulate a melanoma. Nonpigmented adenocarcinoma of the RPE can pose serious diagnostic dilemma. FNAB is helpful in such circumstances. One such case of adenocarcinoma has been reported, where FNAB was

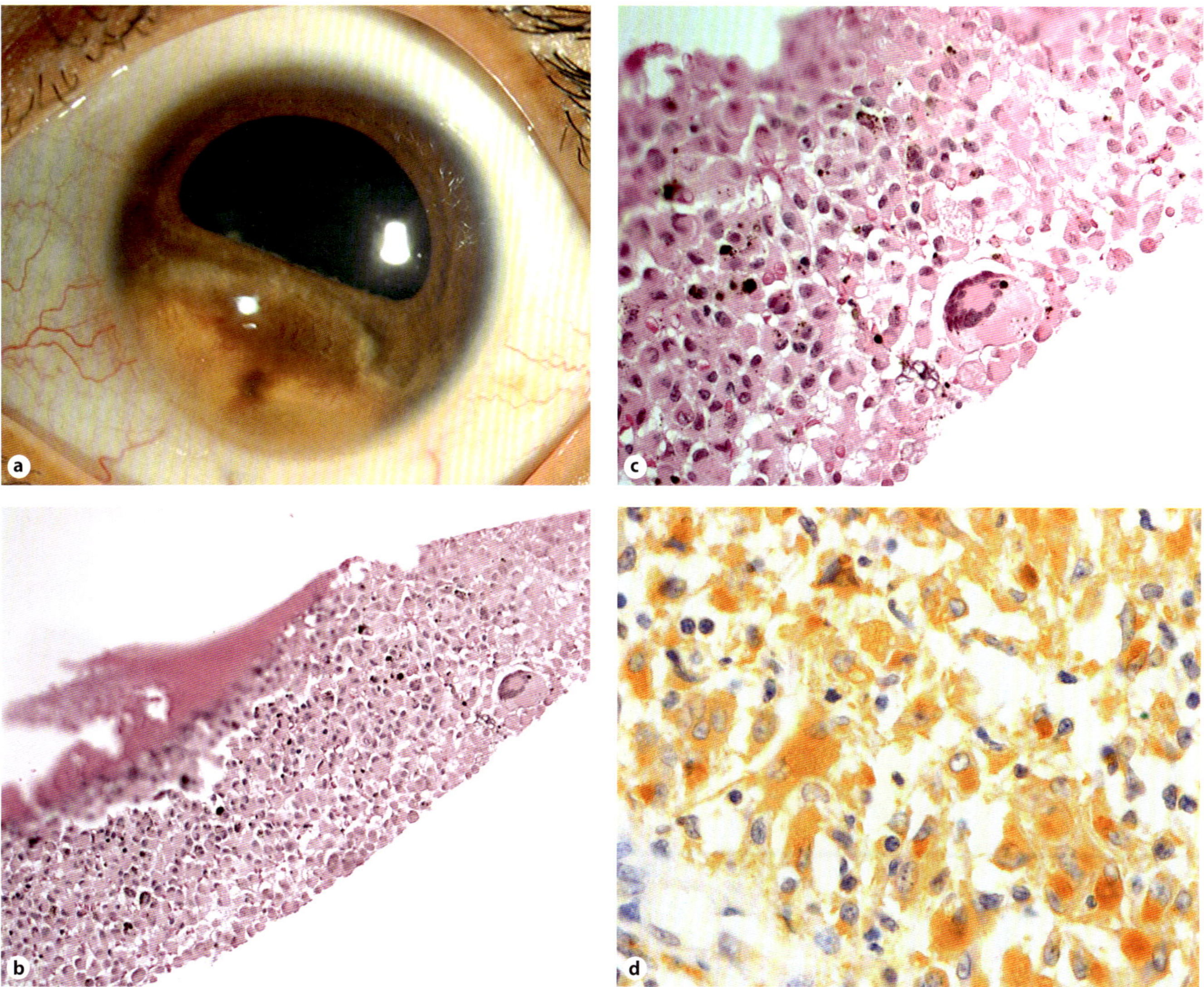

Fig. 5. Juvenile xanthogranuloma. Anterior segment photograph showing the predominant involvement of the iris (**a**). An FNAB sample has cellular aggregates of histiocytes including foamy histiocytes (**b**, hematoxylin-eosin, ×200) and the typical multinucleated giant cells or Touton giant cells (**c**, hematoxylin-eosin, ×400). CD68 immunostain positivity is seen in some of the larger cells confirming their histiocytic lineage (**d**).

performed because of progressive growth and visual loss [33]. Cytology showed a cluster of cells that were immunoreactive to cytokeratin suggesting a malignant tumor of the RPE. Nodular tumors can also develop from areas of focal hyperplasia of the RPE. Shields et al. [34] have reported 2 such cases, one arising from RPE hyperplasia at the site of laser treatment for central serous retinopathy and the other from RPE hyperplasia at the site of an inflammatory scar. Though the cytopathology in these cases was not conclusive, it did show scant round cells with large spherical pigment granules that were larger than those ordinarily seen in choroidal melanoma [34].

Retinal Astrocytic Tumors

FNAB is usually not needed in the diagnosis of astrocytic hamartoma; however, in atypical cases it may prove to be a valuable diagnostic adjunct [35, 36]. Cytopathology of the FNAB specimen would show characteristic spindle cells with immunohistochemical staining with glial fibrillary acidic protein showing cytoplasmic staining for glial cells and no immunoreactivity to cytokeratin (fig. 7) [36]. Rarely, pigmented variants of acquired retinal astrocytoma may simulate a choroidal melanoma or epithelioma of the RPE. FNAB in such circumstances can be helpful in establishing

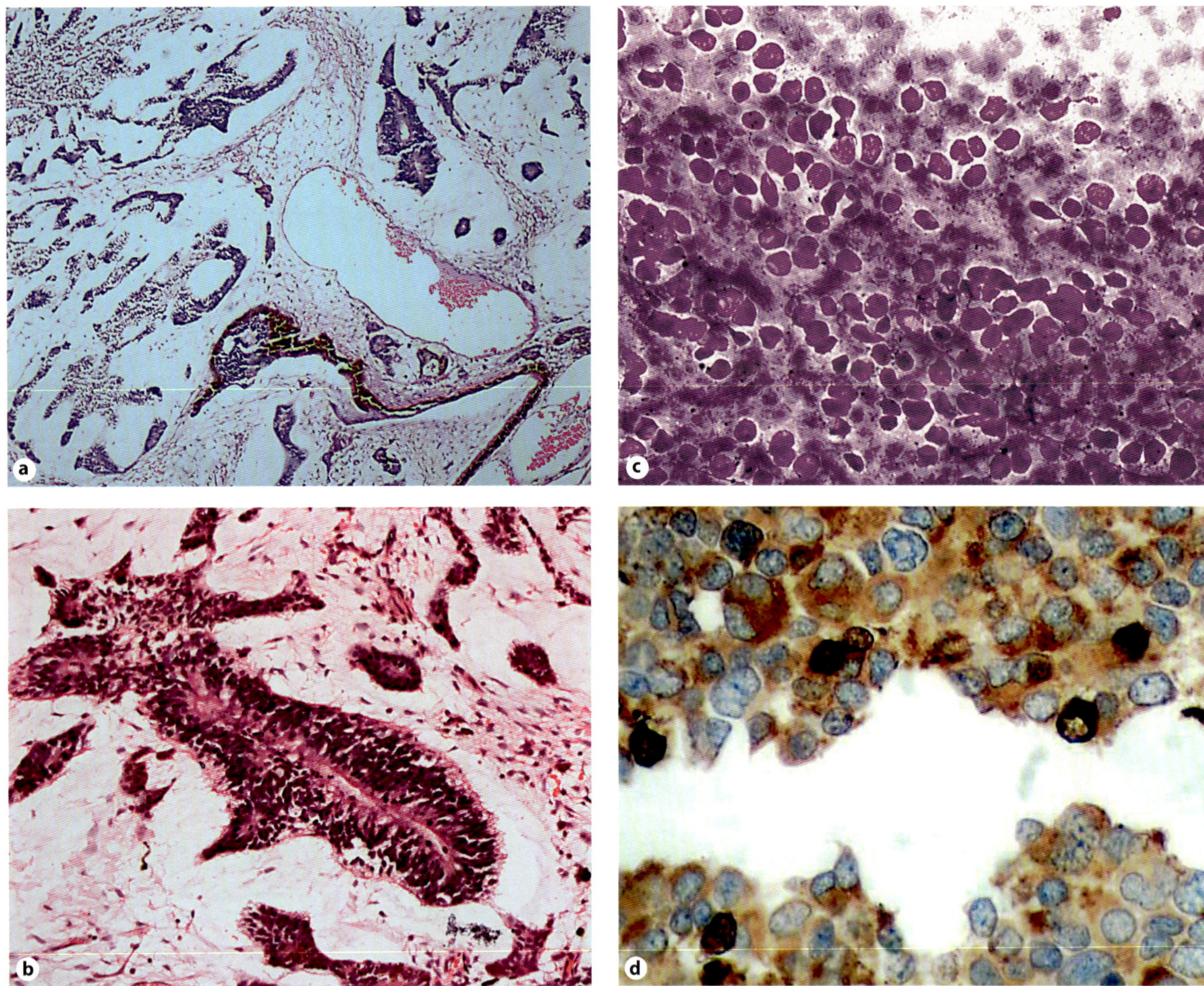

Fig. 6. Medulloepithelioma characterized by primitive neuroepithelial tubules surrounded by variably cellular connective tissue. Hematoxylin-eosin (**a**, **b**). Cellular smear showing a monomorphic sample of cells without appreciable cytoplasm (**c**, Diff-Quik. ×400). Immunohistochemistry with neuron-specific enolase positivity. (**d**, ×400).

the diagnosis. Cytopathology would demonstrate spindle cells with round to ovoid nuclei and glial fibrillary acidic protein positivity; however, melanoma-specific antigen HMB45 and epithelial markers would be negative [36].

Limitations

One of the major limitations of FNAB is the failure to obtain sufficient cytological material to allow the cytopathologist to render a reliable diagnosis. Adequate material for cytological diagnosis was obtained in 88% of patients (140/159) in the series of Shields et al. [1] and 65% (22/34) in that of Augsburger et al. [37]. Factors that may influence this major limitation include the gauge of the needle used and the tumor type and thickness. Most authors prefer a 25-gauge needle [2, 5, 37, 38] while some prefer a 30-gauge needle for the transscleral route and a 27-gauge needle for the transvitreal approach [39, 40]. Poor sample quality can be due to delay in processing, which can be addressed by immediate processing of the specimen in the operating room by the cytopathologist [13, 41–43]. Solid compact tumors composed of strongly cohesive cells yield less material [37]. It is essential to consider the tumor thickness as

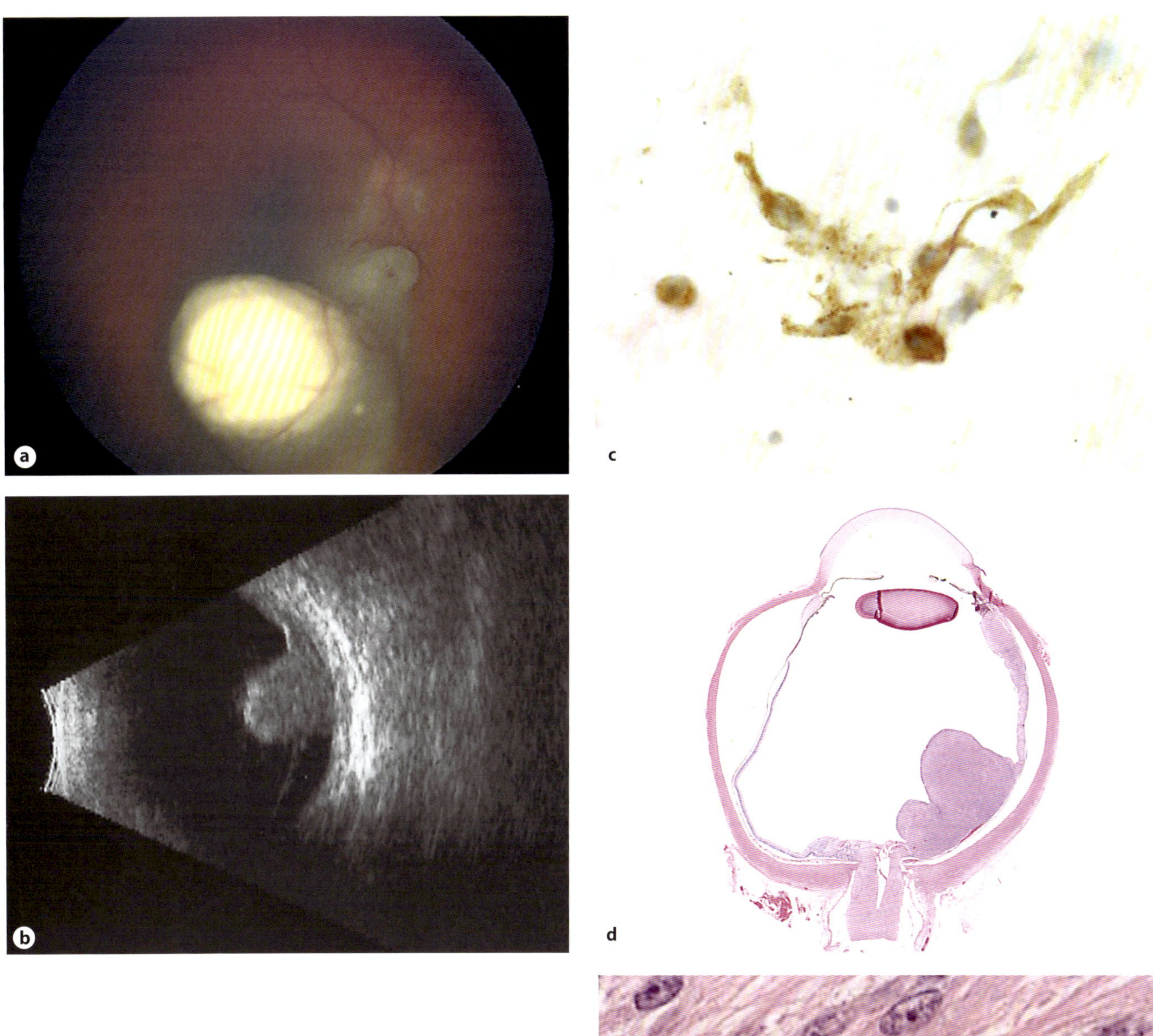

Fig. 7. Astrocytoma. A 5-year-old boy with a multilobulated white-gray retinal mass with overlying vitreous seeding (**a**). Ocular ultrasound examination showed a mushroom-shaped lesion measuring 9.0 mm in thickness. Note the absence of tumor calcification (**b**). Cytopathological analysis after FNAB revealed slender cells with benign features that stained positively for vimentin and glial fibrillary acidic protein, consistent with retinal astrocytoma. Progressive tumor growth prompted enucleation (**c**). The gross specimen contained a homogeneous multilobulated retinal mass without optic nerve invasion (**d**). Histopathological analysis revealed large glial cells with fibrillar cytoplasm and absence of mitotic figures (**e**). Reproduced with permission from Cohen et al. [36].

an important limitation, more so in retinal tumors. Cohen et al. [44] and later Augsburger et al. [37] confirmed the significance of tumor thickness. FNAB is expected to give useful information in lesions more than 3 mm thick and can be often unreliable in lesions <2 mm thick. It is worth emphasizing that while a positive FNAB may be conclusive, a negative result does not exclude a diagnosis [2]. Obtaining a representative sample is therefore the key to an accurate result [45].

Complications

Complications of FNAB include local hemorrhage at the site of entrance in virtually all cases, which can be easily controlled and causes no additional visual impairment. Sometimes significant subretinal and vitreous hemorrhage may occur. Other complications including retinal detachment, tumor seeding, cataract and endophthalmitis are rare [2].

Conclusions

There have been considerable advances in the use and interpretation of noninvasive diagnostic modalities for intraocular tumors. Despite these developments, there are certain atypical cases that defy a clinical diagnosis. In such difficult situations, a carefully considered FNAB may be a useful clinical adjunct. FNAB should be ideally avoided in retinoblastoma unless there is an extreme difficulty in diagnosis – it is never to be used just to 'confirm' an obvious clinical diagnosis. An experienced and qualified cytopathologist armed with the knowledge of ocular histology and intraocular tumor pathology is mandatory for accurate reporting of FNAB of retinal tumors. It is equally essential for the ophthalmologist to communicate with the cytopathologist, provide all the relevant clinical information and discuss the differential diagnosis so that adequate preparation is done for immunohistochemical studies.

References

1 Shields JA, Shields CL, Ehya H, Eagle RC Jr, De Potter P: Fine-needle aspiration biopsy of suspected intraocular tumors: the 1992 Urwick lecture. Ophthalmology 1993;100:1677–1684.

2 Eide N, Walaas L: Fine-needle aspiration biopsy and other biopsies in suspected intraocular malignant disease: a review. Acta Ophthalmol 2009;87:588–601.

3 Char DH, Miller TR: Fine needle biopsy in retinoblastoma. Am J Ophthalmol 1984;97:686–690.

4 Karcioglu ZA: Fine needle aspiration biopsy (FNAB) for retinoblastoma. Retina 2002;22:707–710.

5 Coman DR: Adhesiveness and stickiness: two independent properties of the cell surface. Cancer Res 1961;21:1436–1438.

6 Robertson DM: Fine-needle biopsy and retinoblastoma. Ophthalmology 1997;104:567–568.

7 Henkes HE, Manschot WA: The danger of diagnostic biopsy in eyes suspected of an intraocular tumour. Ophthalmologica 1963;145:467–469.

8 Makley TA Jr: Biopsy of intraocular lesions. Am J Ophthalmol 1967;64(suppl):591–599.

9 Karcioglu ZA, Gordon RA, Karcioglu GL: Tumor seeding in ocular fine needle aspiration biopsy. Ophthalmology 1985;92:1763–1767.

10 Ryd W, Hagmar B, Eriksson O: Local tumour cell seeding by fine-needle aspiration biopsy: a semiquantitative study. Acta Pathol Microbiol Immunol Scand A 1983;91:17–21.

11 Honavar SG, Rajeev B: Needle tract tumor cell seeding following fine needle aspiration biopsy for retinoblastoma. Invest Ophthalmol Vis Sci 1998;39:S658.

12 Augsburger JJ, Shields JA, Folberg R, Lang W, O'Hara BJ, Claricci JD: Fine needle aspiration biopsy in the diagnosis of intraocular cancer: cytologic-histologic correlations. Ophthalmology 1985;92:39–49.

13 Eide N, Syrdalen P, Walaas L, Hagmar B: Fine needle aspiration biopsy in selecting treatment for inconclusive intraocular disease. Acta Ophthalmol Scand 1999;77:448–452.

14 O'Hara BJ, Ehya H, Shields JA, Augsburger JJ, Shields CL, Eagle RC Jr: Fine needle aspiration biopsy in pediatric ophthalmic tumors and pseudotumors. Acta Cytol 1993;37:125–130.

15 Crosby MB, Hubbard GB, Gallie BL, Grossniklaus HE: Anterior diffuse retinoblastoma: mutational analysis and immunofluorescence staining. Arch Pathol Lab Med 2009;133:1215–1218.

16 Rosenthal DL, Mandel DB, Glasgow BJ: Eye; in Bibbo M (ed): Comprehensive Cytopathology. Philadelphia, Saunders, 1991, pp 484–501.

17 Akhtar M, Ali MA, Sabbah R, Sackey K, Bakry M: Aspiration cytology of retinoblastoma: light and electron microscopic correlations. Diagn Cytopathol 1988;4:306–311.

18 Scroggs MW, Johnston WW, Klintworth GK: Intraocular tumors: a cytopathologic study. Acta Cytol 1990;34:401–408.

19 Alio J, Ludena M, Millan A, Caballero V, Guinaldo V: Ultrastructural study of a retinoma by intraocular fine-needle aspiration biopsy. Ophthalmologica 1988;196:192–199.

20 Shields JA, Shields CL, Honavar SG, Demirci H: Clinical variations and complications of Coats disease in 150 cases: the 2000 Sanford Gifford memorial lecture. Am J Ophthalmol 2001;131:561–571.

21 Shields JA, Shields CL: Differentiation of Coats' disease and retinoblastoma. J Pediatr Ophthalmol Strabismus 2001;38:262–266, quiz 302–263.

22 Glasgow BJ, Foos RY: Abnormalities of Retina. Oxford, Butterworth-Heinemann, 1993.

23 Werner JC, Ross RD, Green WR, Watts JC: Pars plana vitrectomy and subretinal surgery for ocular toxocariasis. Arch Ophthalmol 1999;117:532–534.

24 Shields JA: Ocular toxocariasis: a review. Surv Ophthalmol 1984;28:361–381.

25 De Visser L, Rothova A, de Boer JH, et al: Diagnosis of ocular toxocariasis by establishing intraocular antibody production. Am J Ophthalmol 2008;145:369–374.

26 Shields JA, Parsons HM, Shields CL, Shah P: Lesions simulating retinoblastoma. J Pediatr Ophthalmol Strabismus 1991;28:338–340.

27 Howard GM, Ellsworth RM: Differential diagnosis of retinoblastoma: a statistical survey of 500 children. I. Relative frequency of the lesions which simulate retinoblastoma. Am J Ophthalmol 1965;60:610–618.

28 Shields JA, Shields CL, Eagle RC Jr, Barrett J, De Potter P: Endogenous endophthalmitis simulating retinoblastoma: the 1993 David and Mary Seslen endowment lecture. Retina 1995;15:213–219.

29 De Barge LR, Chan CC, Greenberg SC, McLean IW, Yannuzzi LA, Nussenblatt RB: Chorioretinal, iris, and ciliary body infiltration by juvenile xanthogranuloma masquerading as uveitis. Surv Ophthalmol 1994;39:65–71.
30 Shields JA, Eagle RC Jr, Shields CL, Collins ML, De Potter P: Iris juvenile xanthogranuloma studied by immunohistochemistry and flow cytometry. Ophthalmic Surg Lasers 1997;28:140–144.
31 Shields JA, Eagle RC Jr, Shields CL, De Potter P: Congenital neoplasms of the nonpigmented ciliary epithelium (medulloepithelioma). Ophthalmology 1996;103:1998–2006.
32 Shields JA, Eagle RC Jr, Shields CL, Marcus S, De Potter P, Riegel EM: Fluorescein angiography and ultrasonography of malignant intraocular medulloepithelioma. J Pediatr Ophthalmol Strabismus 1996;33:193–196.
33 Shields JA, Eagle RC Jr, Barr CC, Shields CL, Jones DE: Adenocarcinoma of retinal pigment epithelium arising from a juxtapapillary histoplasmosis scar. Arch Ophthalmol 1994;112:650–653.
34 Shields JA, Shields CL, Slakter J, Wood W, Yannuzzi LA: Locally invasive tumors arising from hyperplasia of the retinal pigment epithelium. Retina 2001;21:487–492.
35 Shields JA, Shields CL, Ehya H, Buckley E, De Potter P: Atypical retinal astrocytic hamartoma diagnosed by fine-needle biopsy. Ophthalmology 1996;103:949–952.
36 Cohen VM, Shields CL, Furuta M, Shields JA: Vitreous seeding from retinal astrocytoma in three cases. Retina 2008;28:884–888.
37 Augsburger JJ, Correa ZM, Schneider S, et al: Diagnostic transvitreal fine-needle aspiration biopsy of small melanocytic choroidal tumors in nevus versus melanoma category. Trans Am Ophthalmol Soc 2002;100:225–232, discussion 232.
38 Midena E, Segato T, Piermarocchi S, Boccato P: Fine needle aspiration biopsy in ophthalmology. Surv Ophthalmol 1985;29:410–422.
39 Shields CL, Ganguly A, Materin MA, et al: Chromosome 3 analysis of uveal melanoma using fine-needle aspiration biopsy at the time of plaque radiotherapy in 140 consecutive cases: the Deborah Iverson, MD, lectureship. Arch Ophthalmol 2007;125:1017–1024.
40 Young TA, Burgess BL, Rao NP, Glasgow BJ, Straatsma BR: Transscleral fine-needle aspiration biopsy of macular choroidal melanoma. Am J Ophthalmol 2008;145:297–302.
41 Char DH, Miller T: Accuracy of presumed uveal melanoma diagnosis before alternative therapy. Br J Ophthalmol 1995;79:692–696.
42 Faulkner-Jones BE, Foster WJ, Harbour JW, Smith ME, Davila RM: Fine needle aspiration biopsy with adjunct immunohistochemistry in intraocular tumor management. Acta Cytol 2005;49:297–308.
43 Young TA, Burgess BL, Rao NP, Gorin MB, Straatsma BR: High-density genome array is superior to fluorescence in-situ hybridization analysis of monosomy 3 in choroidal melanoma fine needle aspiration biopsy. Mol Vis 2007;13:2328–2333.
44 Cohen VM, Dinakaran S, Parsons MA, Rennie IG: Transvitreal fine needle aspiration biopsy: the influence of intraocular lesion size on diagnostic biopsy result. Eye (Lond) 2001;15:143–147.
45 Robertson DM: Cytogenetics in the management of uveal melanoma: are we there yet? Arch Ophthalmol 2008;126:409–410.

Arun D. Singh, MD, Professor of Ophthalmology
Director, Department of Ophthalmic Oncology, Cole Eye Institute, Cleveland Clinic Foundation
9500 Euclid Avenue
Cleveland, OH 44195 (USA)
Tel. +1 216 445 9479, E-Mail singha@ccf.org

Biscotti CV, Singh AD (eds): FNA Cytology of Ophthalmic Tumors.
Monogr Clin Cytol. Basel, Karger 2012, vol 21, pp 82–89

Fine Needle Aspiration Cytology in Orbital Tumors

Stefan Seregard[a] · Edneia Tani[b]

[a]St. Eriks Eye Hospital, Karolinska Institutet, and [b]Department of Pathology and Cytology, Karolinska University Hospital Solna, Karolinska Institutet, Stockholm, Sweden

The orbit largely resembles a pyramid with the apex located deep facing the orbital foramen and the base situated at the surface of the eye. Although the bony walls effectively obstruct any attempts to enter a needle, the deep orbit may be accessed at the base of the pyramid. However, the globe blocks most of this entrance leaving only the space along the orbital rim accessible for fine needle aspiration (FNA). This makes FNA more challenging, and deep lesions will require precise positioning of the needle in terms of angle and depth.

Furthermore, the orbit is traversed by numerous delicate structures including small peripheral nerves and blood vessels. Adipose tissue is immaculately arranged in small compartments separated by minute septae and tends to obscure visibility. Irrespectively of whether FNA is to be performed by an ophthalmologist, cytopathologist or an interventional radiologist, knowledge of orbital anatomy is paramount. Although this would suggest that the orbit is less suited for FNA, the small 27-gauge (0.45-mm) diameter of the needle minimizes morbidity, and the path to deeper lesions may be guided by ultrasound or computerized tomography (CT) imaging. Core needle biopsies may provide more material, but at the expense of a much higher rate of complications and are rarely used in the orbit. The use of supplementary techniques like immunocytochemistry and flow cytometry and more recently the advent of molecular genetic workup have markedly improved diagnostic accuracy. While earlier series report a correct diagnosis in 75–88% of orbital FNA biopsies, more recent data using immunocytochemistry and other techniques indicate a diagnostic accuracy of up to 99% [1].

In Stockholm, FNA biopsy is currently used for a wide range of tumors in all parts of the body. Refined FNA in cancer dates back to the early 1960s and has been used in orbital tumors since the 1970s in Stockholm. For orbital diseases, this has evolved into a team effort including dedicated ophthalmologists, cytopathologists and more recently interventional radiologists. Currently, FNA cytology is the mainstay of morphological diagnosis for orbital tumors in Stockholm, rarely being replaced as the primary procedure by open biopsy. Below there are comments on some of the specifics of FNA performed in more frequent tumors such as those of the lacrimal gland, lymphocytic tumors and tumors metastatic to the orbit. We have not addressed the less frequent soft tissue tumors and optic nerve tumors.

Technique

Initially, the FNAs in our setting were performed by an ophthalmologist with a cytopathologist present. Currently, the cytopathologist performs the FNA for the majority of superficial, usually palpable, lesions, and the interventional radiologist undertakes the CT-guided FNA biopsies for nonpalpable more posterior tumors together with the cytopathologist who takes care of the sample and after quick staining evaluates the representativity of the material. The role of the ophthalmologist has evolved into one of defining appropriate cases for biopsy and to provide tentative diagnoses. We advise cessation of aspirin or nonsteroidal anti-inflammatory drugs 1 week before FNA of deeper orbital lesions. Similarly, anticoagulant therapy is usually

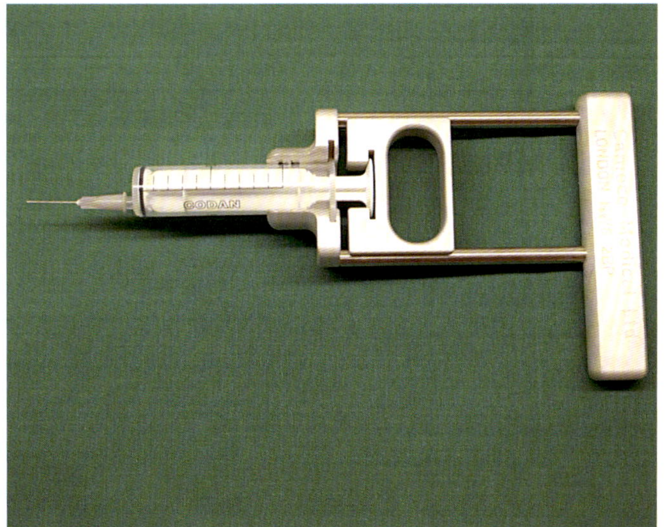

Fig. 1. Ten-ml syringe holder pistol with a 27-gauge needle.

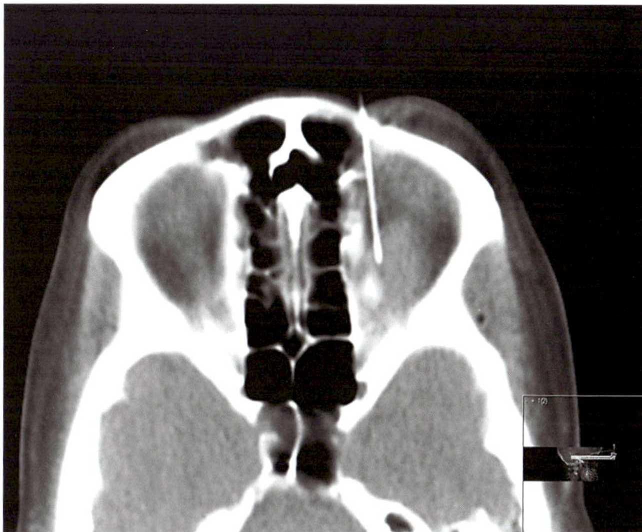

Fig. 2. A 3-mm CT transaxial section through the upper orbit. FNA is used for a nonpalpable lesion in the posterior part of the orbit during verification of the needle position.

discontinued a few days before CT-guided orbital FNA biopsy. The procedure is performed on a strictly outpatient basis with the patient remaining for observation up to 1 h after FNA.

For the palpable lesions we use a thin 27-gauge (0.45-mm) needle fitted to a 10-ml syringe in a one-hand grip syringe holder pistol (fig. 1). When the needle is in the target, suction is applied while the needle is moved back and forth through the lesion. Nonpalpable lesions are biopsied with a 25-gauge (0.53-mm) needle with a stylet and CT guidance. When the needle is in the lesion (fig. 2), the stylet is removed, and the syringe with the holder is attached to apply suction for sampling.

Processing/Staining

Part of the aspirate is ejected onto a glass slide to make a smear for morphological examination. The air-dried smear is stained with May-Grünwald-Giemsa and immediately assessed for adequacy of the sample. The remaining material can be rinsed in 1.5 ml phosphate-buffered saline to provide a cell suspension for further ancillary techniques such as flow cytometry, immunostaining on cytospin preparations and cytogenetic analysis. When necessary, repeat passes may be performed (though usually not more than 2–3 passes). More details of the general aspects of the FNA technique have been published elsewhere [2].

Immunohistochemistry
Immunocytochemical analysis for markers with nuclear staining are performed on smears with an immunoperoxidase technique. Cytospin preparations are used for membrane and cytoplasmic staining with a 3-step alkaline phosphatase technique as described previously [3].

Immunophenotyping
To confirm monoclonality and diagnose lymphoma, we use immunocytochemistry and/or flow cytometry. Flow cytometry is best used for a fresh cell suspension and may be performed in hours to detect multiple antigens at the same time. In contrast, immunocytochemistry detects one antigen for each staining and may use archival air-dried cytospins. Special protocols have been developed for the study of orbital lymphoproliferative disease [4].

Genotyping
Cytogenetic testing now available to detect chromosomal translocations specific for various orbital tumors has been elaborated on elsewhere [5]. Other techniques now becoming more frequent include karyotyping, fluorescence in situ hybridization, Southern blot hybridization and polymerase chain reaction to detect chromosomal translocations, rearrangements of the immunoglobulin heavy chain genes and T-cell receptor genes. It is beyond the scope of this text to detail all the techniques available and the characteristics of various subtypes of orbital lymphoma.

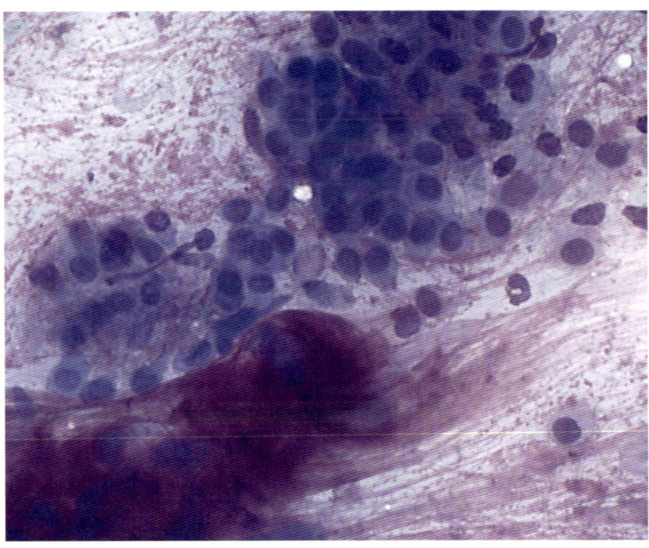

Fig. 3. Lacrimal gland pleomorphic adenoma. The FNA smear shows monomorphic myoepithelial cells and a pinkish fibrillary chondromyxoid stroma.

Clinical Indications

Lacrimal Fossa Lesions

Most space-occupying lesions of the lacrimal fossa arise from the lacrimal gland. Although most lacrimal gland lesions are inflammatory, the majority of lesions requiring a cytological or histopathological diagnosis are neoplastic. The reported frequency of neoplastic lesions of the lacrimal gland differs, but in our experience approximately some two thirds of these lesions are epithelial, e.g. pleomorphic adenoma (fig. 3), adenoid cystic adenocarcinoma (fig. 4) and adenocarcinoma, and one third lymphocytic, e.g. lymphoma and lymphocytic hyperplasia [6].

Management depends on diagnosis as epithelial lesions are typically excised and lymphocytic lesions are often treated by radiotherapy and/or chemotherapy sometimes combined with oral corticosteroids. Unfortunately, a reliable diagnosis of neoplastic lacrimal gland lesions can rarely be made solely by clinical examination and imaging studies. Below we will briefly discuss the case for FNA in lacrimal gland tumors.

Lacrimal gland tumors are notoriously difficult to diagnose by clinical and radiological features only, and misdiagnosis may occur in 20% or more of presumed lacrimal gland pleomorphic adenoma (LGPA) [7]. Incisional biopsies of lacrimal gland lesions have been discouraged for fear that violation of the thin pseudocapsule surrounding LGPA may cause tumor seeding. Although a recent review suggested that there is no proof that incisional biopsy increases the risk for orbital recurrence [8], there are abundant anecdotal data of patients requiring orbital exenteration because of multifocal LGPA seeded at the time of previous surgery. Until this issue has been resolved, FNA remains a viable option in the diagnosis of LGPA [7, 9]. Notably, we used FNA cytology to reliably diagnose LGPA in 15/15 patients without any recurrence after a median follow-up of 67 months (range: 11–135 months) [9].

The salivary glands are structured in much the same way as the lacrimal gland, and much more data from FNA cytology are available for salivary gland tumors. Recently, a structured review based on 16 studies of salivary gland tumors reported an impressive 95 and 80% concordance between cytological analysis and subsequent histopathological studies in 1,275 benign tumors and 484 malignant tumors, respectively [10]. The clinician should be wary; we have experienced a patient with an adenoid cystic carcinoma of the lacrimal gland misdiagnosed elsewhere as LGPA based on FNA cytology.

Another advantage of cytopathology in lacrimal gland tumors is that FNA sampling may easily distinguish lymphoproliferative lesions from epithelial tumors. Lymphoproliferative tumors may then be subdivided by ancillary techniques like immunocytochemistry and flow cytometry as discussed in the next section.

Lymphoproliferative Tumors

The orbit may harbor both benign (lymphocytic hyperplasia) and malignant (lymphoma) lymphoproliferative disase. Orbital lymphoma is the most common orbital malignancy, and there is some evidence that the incidence is rising. Typically, orbital lymphoma arises from the lacrimal gland or the extraocular muscles, but may also present as a more diffuse mass molding to surrounding tissue (like the globe) and slowly pushing it away. Most orbital lymphomas arise in the anterior or middle orbit and are often palpable, rendering them easily accessible to FNA biopsy. When a monoclonal origin cannot be proven, a diagnosis of lymphocytic hyperplasia is usually made. Some patients with lymphocytic hyperplasia of the orbit will later experience recurrence from biopsy-proven orbital lymphoma.

Surprisingly, even recent papers sometimes advise against needle biopsies and advocate open sky biopsy to secure enough tissue for diagnosis [11]. In contrast, our experience indicates that FNA biopsy followed by cytomorphological assessment and ancillary techniques like immunocytochemistry and/or flow cytometry are almost always sufficient for diagnosis. An FNA setting with a cytopathologist present to immediately make a tentative diagnosis by morphology and

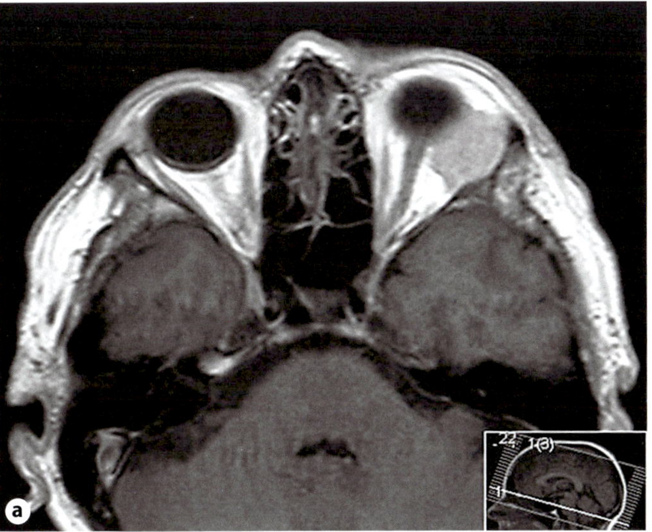

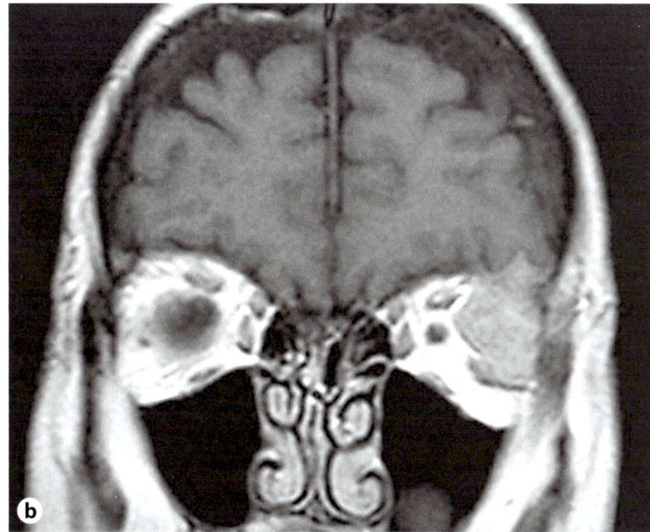

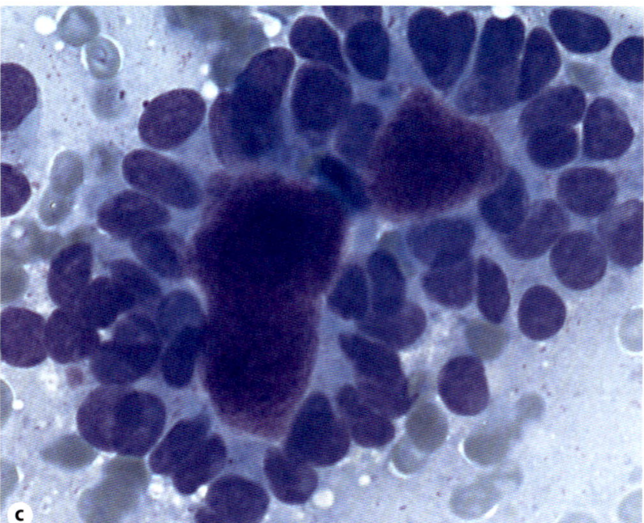

Fig. 4. Lacrimal gland adenoid cystic carcinoma. A 3-mm contrast-enhanced transaxial (**a**) and coronal (**b**) magnetic resonance slice shows a solid unspecific mass in the left orbit. The FNA smear features basaloid tumor cells arranged in rosette-like formations surrounding homogeneous round pink globules (**c**, May-Grünwald-Giemsa stain).

then securing enough cells for ancillary tests (if required by additional needle passes) saves the patient an operating procedure. In our hands, this technique confirmed lymphoma in 35/37 cases with cytomorphologically suspect orbital lymphoma (fig. 5). One of the 2 remaining patients was diagnosed with so-called orbital pseudotumor (idiopathic orbital inflammation) on open biopsy, and the other patient later had a local relapse with FNA-proven lymphoma [1].

Metastatic Lesions

Primary breast carcinoma is the most common source of orbital metastases, but a wide variety of malignant tumors may disseminate to the orbit. Most patients have a history of malignant disease elsewhere, but orbital metastases may be the first sign of extraorbital malignant disease. The classic mode of presentation for orbital metastases is a circumscribed mass confined to an extraocular muscle, though the pattern may sometimes be more diffuse.

Immunocytochemistry has shown to be a helpful adjunct to cytomorphology when tracing the origin of malignant cells. Many primary tumors show characteristic immunoreactivity for one or more antigens, and the same profile is usually repeated in the metastases. Judicial use of an appropriate panel of monoclonal antibodies may suggest a source of origin of metastases, even when the site of the primary tumor is unknown (fig. 6).

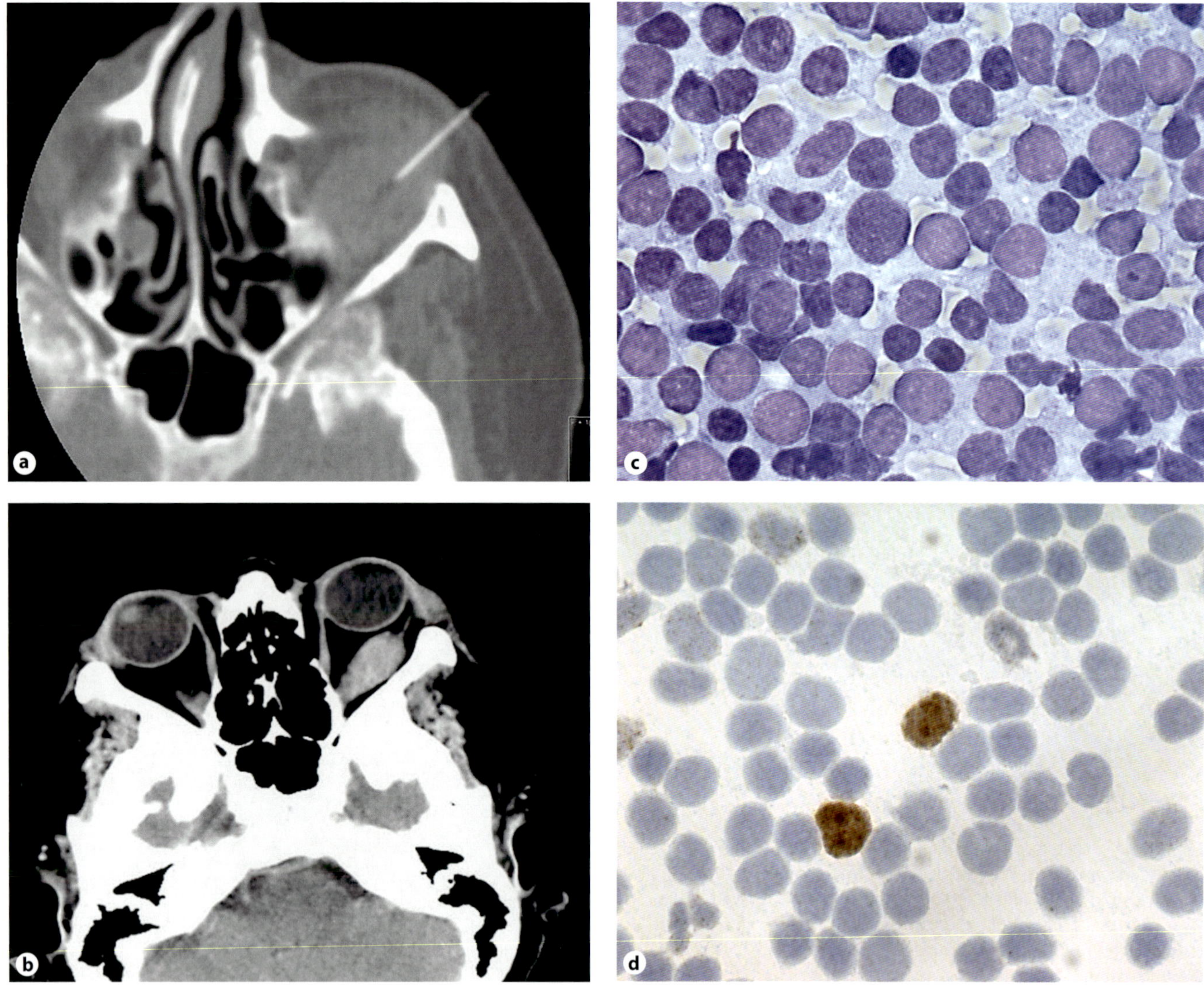

Fig. 5. Mantle cell lymphoma of the orbit. A CT-guided FNA of an orbital mass (**a**). A 2-mm transaxial contrast-enhanced CT section shows a solid vascularized tumor laterally in the orbit (**b**). The FNA smear shows medium-sized lymphoid cells with scanty round or irregular nuclear cytoplasm (**c**, May-Grünwald-Giemsa stain). The Ki-67-stained smear shows 2 proliferating tumor cells with distinct nuclear staining. Immunoperoxidase stain (**d**).

Limitations

Clearly, the use of FNA will provide less material for analysis than sampling by incisional or excisional biopsy (or by a core needle biopsy). This need not be a shortcoming as FNA samples may be monitored for adequacy in the operating room and repeat passes made as required. However, as an FNA will yield disrupted cells and small clusters of cells, the tissue structure (histology) provided by an open biopsy is lost. To some extent, this disadvantage has been overcome with the advent of techniques like immunocytochemistry and flow cytometry, which are based on the studies of single cells.

Some tumors are less suited for FNA, in particular those that are made up by cells identical to the ones normally appearing in the orbit. One of the most frequent orbital tumors is the so-called cavernous hemangioma, a vascular malformation (hamartoma) typically occurring in the intraconal space. An FNA biopsy of a cavernous hemangioma will typically yield endothelial cells, fibroblasts and abundant erythrocytes. As there are no unique

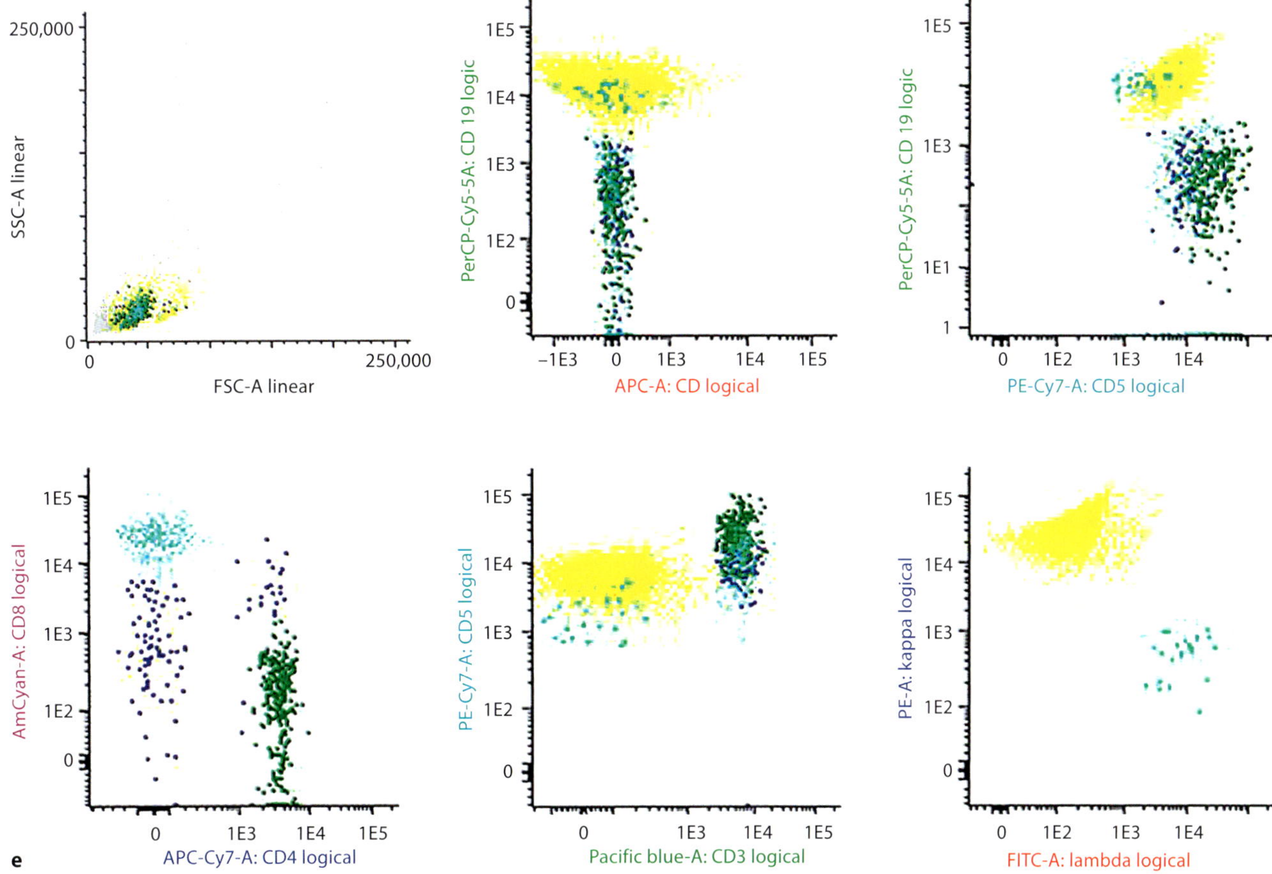

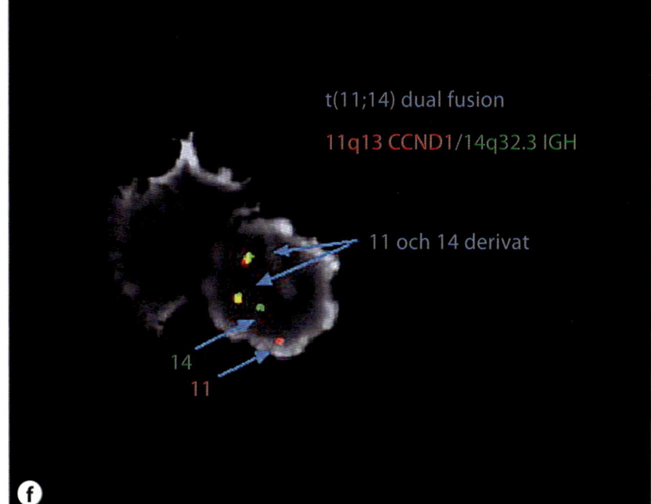

Fig. 5. Flow cytometry immunophenotyping with 8-color cytometry (**e**). The upper left plot shows a forward scatter/side scatter image of the sample with small, nongranulated cells. The upper middle plot shows CD19-positive B cells (yellow and blue dots) and CD3-positive T cells (green and cyan dots). The upper right plot shows that CD4-positive T cells (green dots) are more numerous than CD8-positive T cells (cyan dots). The lower left plot shows that CD19-positive B cells are dimly CD5 positive and T cells are brighter CD5 positive. The lower middle plot illustrates that both B cells and T cells are negative for CD10. The lower right plot shows monoclonal κ-positive B cells (yellow dots) and λ-positive B cells (blue dots). Interphase fluorescence in situ hybridization on tumor cell (**f**, Vysis LSI IgH/CCNDI dual-color, dual-fusion translocation probe) detecting the translocation t(11;14)(q13;q32). In a normal cell, 2 red (CCNDI) and 2 green (IgH) signals are identified (not shown). In the tumor cell, the translocation splits the 2 genes and creates 2 red/green fusion signals. Courtesy of E. Blennow, MD, Clinical Genetics Department, Karolinska University Hospital Solna.

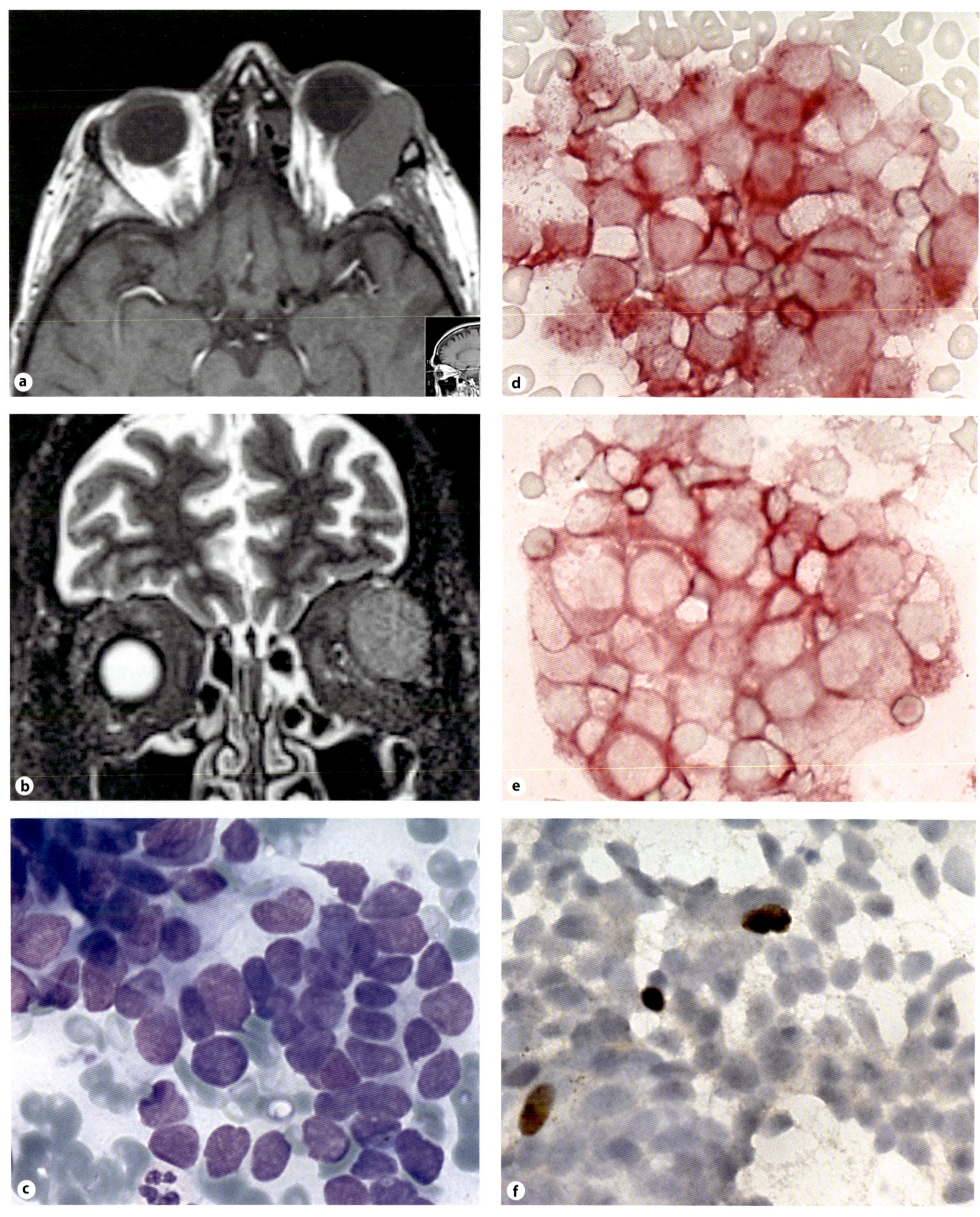
a
b
c
d
e
f

cytomorphological features and a similar cytological finding could result from an accidental hemorrhage, the diagnosis would remain in doubt even after a successful FNA. However, cavernous hemangioma of the orbit can usually be characterized by CT and/or magnetic resonance imaging without the need for FNA. Also, an FNA biopsy of a lymphatic or venous-lymphatic malformation may cause extensive orbital hemorrhage if the delicate blood vessels within the septae separating the larger vascular spaces are ruptured. This remains one of the dreaded (if rare) complications of FNA biopsy of orbital tumors.

Optic nerve tumors are infrequently sampled by FNA; the obvious limitation in optic nerve meningioma is the proximity to the optic nerve proper, and both meningioma and glioma of the optic nerve are often readily diagnosed by neuroradiological imaging. Tumors of the orbital apex are also less often diagnosed by FNA cytology because of fear of damaging the delicate structures crowding in the orbital apex. In fact, the only serious adverse effect (transient visual loss) we have experienced after many hundreds of orbital FNA biopsies was in a patient with a small tumor lodged deep in the orbital apex.

Conclusions

Orbital FNA cytology has some limitations as indicated above but has the potential, when used at the discretion of an experienced team, to replace most open biopsies for orbital tumors. Many of the techniques now used to diagnose and subtype lymphoma and the molecular genetic studies increasingly used to diagnose some of the rarer soft tissue tumors have advanced the possibilities for orbital FNA cytology. Arguably, the skill and training required to perform successful orbital FNA cytology suggest that patients with orbital tumors should be managed by a dedicated referral center.

References

1 Tani E, Seregard S, Rudd G, Söderlund V, Skoog L: Fine-needle aspiration cytology and immunocytochemistry of orbital masses. Diagn Cytopathol 2006;34:1–5.
2 Buley ID, Roskell DE: Fine-needle aspiration cytology in tumour diagnosis: uses and limitations. Clin Oncol 2000;12:166–171.
3 Tani EM, Christensson B, Porwit A, Skoog L: Immunocytochemical analysis and cytomorphological diagnosis on fine needle aspirates of lymphoproliferative diseases. Acta Cytol 1988;32: 209–215.
4 Bradley KT, Arber DA, Brown MS, Chung C-C, Coupland SE, de Baca ME, Ellis DW, Foucar K, Hsi ED, Jaffe ES, Lill MC, McClure SP, Medeiros LJ, Perkins SL, Hussong JW: Protocol for the examination of specimens from patients with hematopoietic neoplasms of the ocular adnexa. Arch Pathol Lab Med 2010;134:336–340.
5 Khong JJ, Moore S, Prabhakaran VC: Genetic testing in orbital tumors. Orbit 2009;28:88–97.
6 Seregard S, Sahlin S: Panorama of orbital space-occupying lesions: the 24-year experience of a referral centre. Acta Ophthalmol Scand 1999;77:91–98.
7 Prabhakaran VC, Cannon PS, McNab A, Davis G, O'Donnell B, Dolman PJ, Ghabrial R, Selva D: Lesions mimicking lacrimal gland adenoma. Br J Ophthalmol 2010;94:1509–1512.
8 Lai T, Prabhakaran VC, Malhotra R, Silva D: Pleomorphic adenoma of the lacrimal gland. is there a role for biopsy? Eye 2009;23:2–6.
9 Kopp ED, Sahlin S, Tani E, Skoog L, Seregard S: Fine-needle aspiration biopsy in lacrimal gland pleomorphic adenoma. Eye 2010;24:386.
10 Colella G, Cannavale R, Flamminio F, Foschini F: Fine-needle aspiration cytology of salivary gland lesions: a systemic review. J Oral Maxillofac Surg 2010;68:2146–2153.
11 Bernardini F, Bazzan M: Lymphoproliferative disease of the orbit. Curr Opin Ophthalmol 2007; 18:398–401.

Stefan Seregard
Department of Ophthalmic Pathology and Oncology
St. Erik's Eye Hospital, Polhemsgatan 50
SE–11282 Stockholm (Sweden)
Tel. +46 86 723 173, E-Mail stefan.seregard@sankterik.se

Fig. 6. Metastasis to the orbit of neuroendocrine carcinoma. A T_1-weighted transaxial (**a**) and coronal (**b**) magnetic resonance image shows a homogeneous mass in the left orbit. The FNA smear shows a cluster of tumor cells with irregular nuclei of varying size and poorly defined scanty cytoplasm (**c**, May-Grünwald-Giemsa stain). The tumor cells are cytokeratin positive (**d**) and chromogranin positive (**e**). Three cells are proliferating as detected by Ki-67 staining of the nuclei (**f**, Immunoperoxidase technique).

Biscotti CV, Singh AD (eds): FNA Cytology of Ophthalmic Tumors.
Monogr Clin Cytol. Basel, Karger 2012, vol 21, pp 90–96

Future of Ophthalmic Fine Needle Aspiration Biopsy

Arun D. Singh[a] · Braeden Dolan[a] · Charles V. Biscotti[b]

[a]Cole Eye Institute and [b]Department of Anatomic Pathology, Cleveland Clinic Foundation, Cleveland, Ohio, USA

It is impossible, if not fraught with danger, to predict the future, for one can easily get it wrong. Nevertheless, there are changes on the horizon that cannot be ignored. The most significant change is the trend towards incorporation of digital technology in the field of pathology. Other innovations include refinement of fine needle aspiration biopsy (FNAB) technique, instrumentation and sample processing. This review includes appraisal of the imminent changes limited to the field of ophthalmic cytology.

Technique and Instrumentations

The techniques for intraocular biopsy vary depending upon the involved tissue (retina, choroid, subretinal space, vitreous) [1, 2], suspected diagnosis, size, location, associated retinal detachment and clarity of the media [3–7]. Since 1979 the technique of ophthalmic FNAB has essentially remained unchanged. However, several innovations have been reported recently.

Needle Modifications

Needles for ophthalmic FNAB are of 25–30 gauge [Chapter 1, this vol., pp. 1–9]. Likelihood of insufficient samples may be lower with a 22-gauge needle [8] than with a higher-gauge (30-gauge) needle [9]. The long bevel of the available needles can limit full entry of the needle tip into a shallow tumor. A prototype needle with a short bevel and millimeter graduations has been designed (fig. 1) [10]. Preliminary data suggest that the aspirate with the prototype needle may be more cellular than with the standard 25-gauge needle [10].

Aspiration Methods

During ophthalmic FNAB, the aspiration force is generated by exerting outward pull on the plunger of the syringe, attached by tubing to the needle. This requires an assistant as both hands of the operating surgeon are occupied with the positioning of the needle. Developed by Intuitive Ophthalmics LLC alongside physicians at the Duke University Eye Center, the 'Syringe Assist Device' allows the physician to comfortably control the motion of the syringe plunger (both during aspiration and injection), with a single hand, without sacrificing stability or precision (fig. 2). In its current form, the device snaps onto a standard, sterile syringe and allows the physician to both inject and aspirate from the tip of the syringe barrel using his or her index finger. The above device is meant to facilitate single-handed injections, aspirations and biopsies specifically for ophthalmic applications.

Indications

At present, prognostic applications exceed the diagnostic applications of ophthalmic FNAB. It is quite likely that this trend will continue, unless techniques for isolating circulating tumor cells are perfected to the level allowing direct morphological confirmation of a circulating tumor cell [11]. Such single-cell genomic studies [12] may permit prognostication based on circulating tumor cells obviating the need

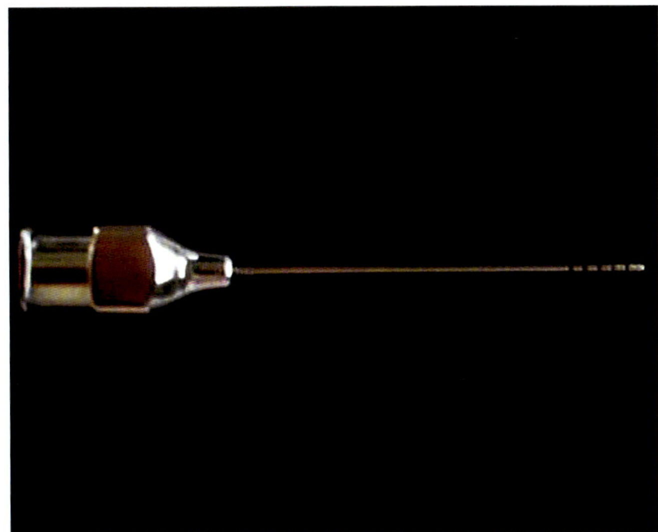

Fig. 1. A prototype 25-gauge needle with short bevel and surface millimeter markings specifically designed for ophthalmic FNAB.

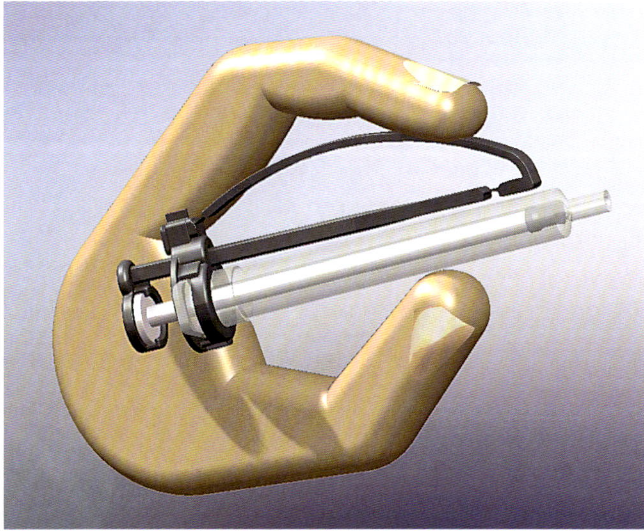

Fig. 2. The Syringe Assist device allows the physician to comfortably control the motion of the syringe plunger (both during aspiration and injection), with a single hand, without sacrificing stability or precision. Courtesy of Intuitive Ophthalmics LLC.

for diagnostic or prognostic biopsy of uveal melanoma [11, 13, 14].

Uveal Metastasis
Diagnosing or excluding the possibility of uveal metastases is one of the most common diagnostic indications for uveal FNAB [Chapter 3, this vol., pp. 17–30; 15, 16]. The diagnosis of uveal metastasis may be uncertain on FNAB because of low cellularity of the sample or because of the highly undifferentiated nature of the tumor. The origin of the primary tumor may not be discernible even with the use of immunohistochemistry. In such cases, the micro-RNA expression pattern (cancer-type-specific micro-RNA signature) can be used for predicting primary sites [17, 18].

Vitreoretinal Lymphoma
Vitrectomy and not FNAB is required to diagnose primary vitreoretinal lymphoma (ophthalmic variant of primary central nervous system lymphoma) as it predominantly manifests as lymphocytic infiltration of the vitreous [Chapter 7, this vol., pp. 61–71; 19]. Because the morphology of an FNAB sample alone is often not sufficient for a definitive diagnosis of lymphoma [20], cytological assessment is often done in conjunction with ancillary studies, such as immunohistochemistry or flow cytometry [21, 22]. The sample may be insufficiently cellular for a definitive morphological diagnosis or ancillary studies [23].

Moreover, differentiation between small lymphocytic lymphomas, metastases and other small round cell tumors (peripheral neuroectodermal tumor, rhabdomyosarcoma and small cell carcinoma) can be challenging in a paucicellular sample wherein immunohistochemistry is not feasible. It is anticipated that in addition to currently used molecular techniques such as fluorescent in situ hybridization and polymerase chain reaction, microarrays and gene profiling will be increasingly used for diagnostic and prognostic subtyping of lymphoma [24].

Melanoma: Prognostic
Uveal FNAB to perform prognostic studies for uveal melanoma is still evolving. The topic is reviewed in detail elsewhere [Chapter 6, this vol., pp. 55–60; 25, 26].

Digital Cytology

The main staple of cytology is the glass slide. Glass slides serve as a means of transportation and preservation of cell samples and allow cytologists instant viewing of the cell sample via a microscope. Some of the limitations of the traditional method are the subjective nature of the interpretation, cumbersome storage and retrieval, and specimen degradation over time. Some of these issues can be solved by incorporating digital technology [27, 28].

Table 1. Digital cytology: pros and contras

Pros	Contras
No physical glass slide to store	Slow scan speeds
Digital archiving	High cost
No specimen degradation or loss of fluorescence	Requires computer skills
Faster retrieval (pattern context-sensitive searches)	Digital alteration of the image impacts interpretation
Quantification	Regulatory and medicolegal issues
Automation	Limited clinical usage (current)
Pattern recognition	
Capable of being 'taught' by user	
Research applications	
Teleconsultation/telediagnosis	

Digital scanning technology has only relatively recently reached the level of sophistication needed in order to be utilized by cytologists, but its applicability is too great to remain unutilized for long (table 1) [29]. The use of high-tech scanners can easily turn glass slides into whole-slide digital images subject to magnification, enhancements, enumeration, morphometry and quantitation. On the issue of archiving, nearly every problem of glass slide archiving can be solved by the introduction of digital archives. Unlike physical matter, pixels do not degrade over time. And with digital archives, cytologists will be able to easily retrieve images that are decades old in order to answer new questions.

Additional possibilities created by digital imaging include digital staining [30], quantification of immunohistochemical stains [31], and rapid fluorescence in situ hybridization analysis [32]. Internet-based systems further extend the applications of digital cytology to telediagnosis and teleconsultation [33, 34], and education, certification and training [35]. One should be aware that digital alterations of the image (alteration of contrast, brightness or color balance) can significantly affect the interpretation of the cytological features and hence the diagnosis [36].

Pattern recognition software has now reached a level of sophistication for clinical usage [37]. There are many versions available, some commercial and some free of charge, produced by different organizations, but they all perform similar functions [38].

Aperio

The biggest name in whole-slide digital scanning and pattern recognition software is Aperio Technologies Inc. (www.Aperio.com). Aperio currently markets 6 scanners differing in slide capacity, magnification capabilities, included viewing software, scanning techniques and speeds, and price. But a scanner is useless without any way of viewing and analyzing the image, so Aperio also produced Image Scope, a viewing program that provides all and more of the functionality of a regular microscope (fig. 3).

The most unique feature offered by Aperio, however, is its pattern recognition software called Genie. In 2007, Aperio secured an exclusive license from Los Alamos National Laboratory for the use of their Genetic Imagery Exploration (Genie Pro) image pattern recognition technology. Genie Pro was used by Los Alamos National Laboratory in satellite imaging for such things as monitoring and analyzing crop health, environmental patterns and damage from natural disasters. Aperio took this technology and decided to apply it to pathology as an add-on to their Spectrum program.

Genie, as defined by Aperio, 'is a general purpose, interactive, adaptive tool for automatically classifying regions and finding regions of interest (such as tumor regions) in large amounts of digital slide data based on a user-defined training set'. Genie utilizes many of the functions of pattern recognition software listed above such as quantifying colocalization, color deconvolution, nuclear size and shape, microvessel analysis, and rare event detection. However, what makes Genie truly unique is its ability to adapt to a user's specifications using genetic programming or 'self-learning'. Users are able to 'teach' Genie to analyze each slide pixel by pixel looking for patterns that the user desires.

A user scans multiple glass slides through an Aperio scanner and is then given a digital image to work with. They can then add these images and general regions of classification to a Genie project in Spectrum. By opening the images in Image Scope, they can annotate the images by classifying regions by different regions (e.g. tumors, stroma). Genie then creates an entirely new algorithm that allows it to identify these regions, according to the user parameters, on new images in the future. So if a cytologist went through the process of teaching Genie to look for a particular pattern, Genie could just apply that same algorithm to study slides.

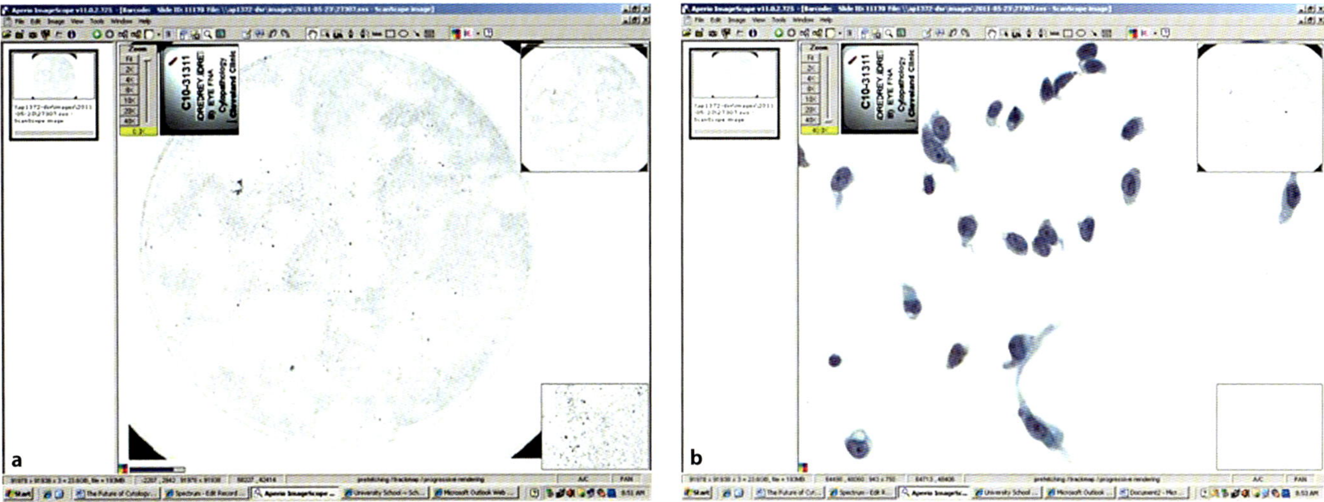

Fig. 3. Screen shot of slide view with Image Scope at the lowest (**a**, ×1) and highest magnifications (**b**, ×40).

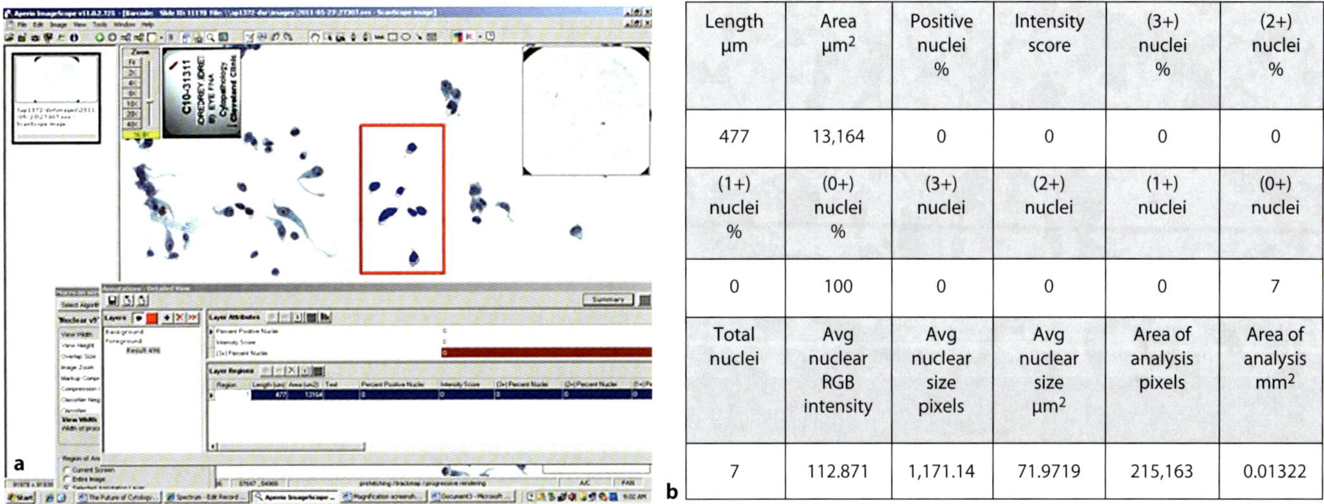

Length µm	Area µm²	Positive nuclei %	Intensity score	(3+) nuclei %	(2+) nuclei %
477	13,164	0	0	0	0
(1+) nuclei %	(0+) nuclei %	(3+) nuclei	(2+) nuclei	(1+) nuclei	(0+) nuclei
0	100	0	0	0	7
Total nuclei	Avg nuclear RGB intensity	Avg nuclear size pixels	Avg nuclear size µm²	Area of analysis pixels	Area of analysis mm²
7	112.871	1,171.14	71.9719	215,163	0.01322

Fig. 4. Screen shot of Image Scope using the Genie Nuclear v9 test (**a**). Data show 43 nuclei with an average size of 89.4962 µm² in the tested region (**b**, annotated by the red rectangle in **a**).

We tested the basics of Genie using a scanned image of a Thinprep slide of an FNAB obtained from a uveal melanoma sample [Chapter 2, this vol., pp. 10–16]. We added annotations to the image of a foreground and background to show Genie which 'patterns' were the cells and what was the background. We then designated a region on the image for Genie to run a nuclear analysis algorithm. By a manual count of the region, we determined there were about 40–45 nuclei in the designated region. Genie Nuclear V9 algorithm provided a count of 43 as well as the average nuclear size and several other parameters (fig. 4).

Cell Profiler

A pattern recognition software called Cell Profiler, developed by the Broad Institute of Harvard and the Massachusetts Institute of Technology, is freely and openly available (www.cellprofiler.org). Cell Profiler works using a system of modules and what are called 'pipelines'. A pipeline is composed

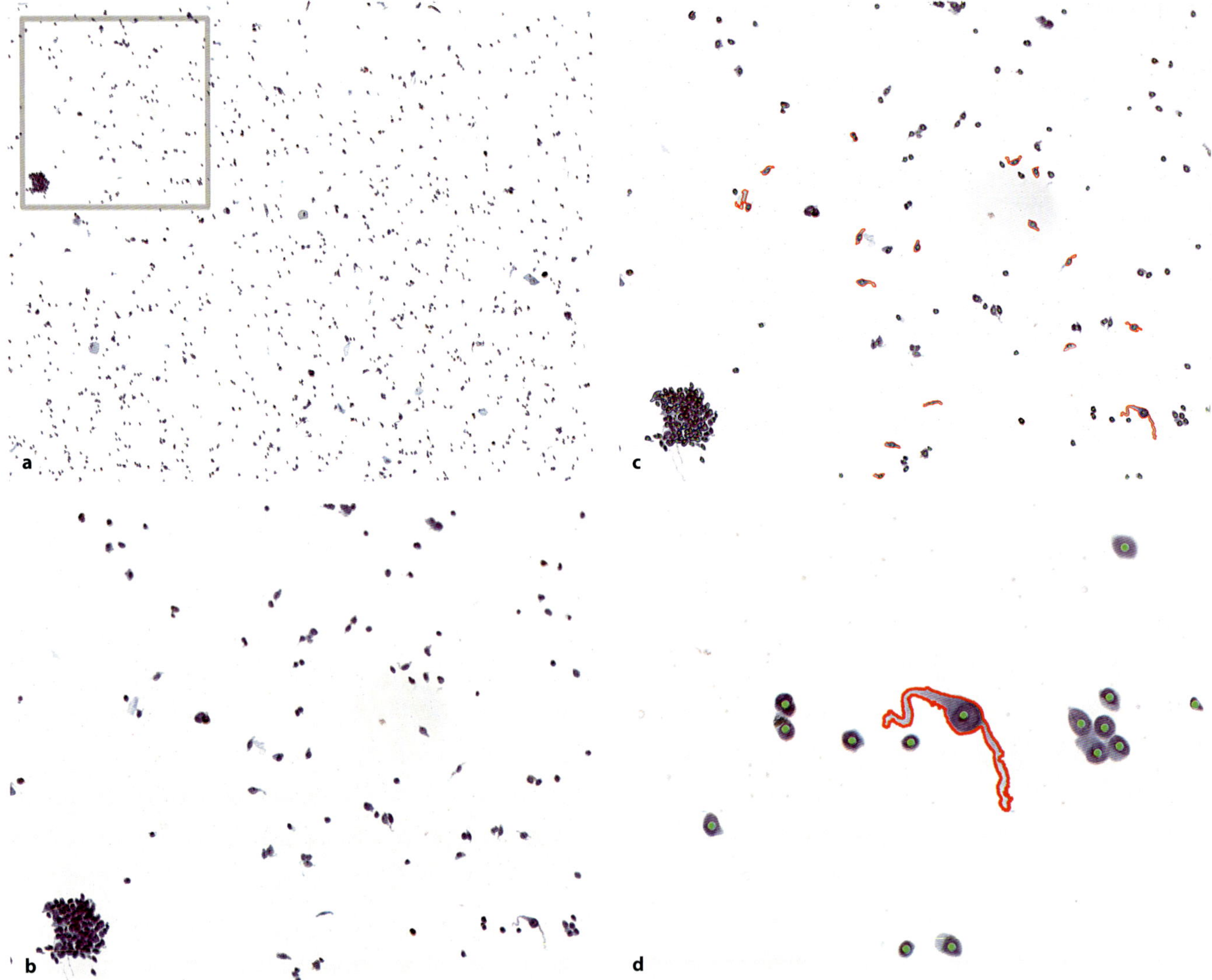

Fig. 5. Cytometric image analysis enabled by Image IQ from an FNAB of uveal melanoma. The Thinprep slide was raster scanned at high resolution using a large field-of-view microscope (×40, 0.185 μm/pixel); 100 image tiles were acquired and stitched together to form a single image (2.96 × 2.22 mm). Low magnification (**a**). High magnification of the area outlined by a square (**b**). This image was subsequently processed and segmented using a variety of customized color space and morphometric filters to generate quantitative data that included total cell counts (220 cells; green dots), detection of cells with spindle-shaped morphology (22 cells; red outlines) and melanin-containing cell counts (7 cells; blue outlines). Low magnification (**c**). High magnification of the area outlined by a square (**d**). Courtesy of Amit Vasanji, PhD, and Nathan Tenley, Image IQ Inc.

of user-selected modules, which are the specific functions Cell Profiler can perform. Users craft their own pipelines by selecting the modules they would like Cell Profiler to run. Modules include e.g. loading images, exporting images, automatic cropping for regions of interest, identifying objects of interest, measuring size, shape and area or counting cells. Thus, Cell Profiler modules are very relatable to Genie functions, but Cell Profiler in its current form does not have the ability to create new algorithms based on user specifications.

Customized Image Analysis (Image IQ)

Due to the infinite variations in image acquisition and staining protocols, quantitative analysis of cytological images using commercially available or open-source software can be challenging in terms of feasibility and precision. Using an extensive library of image-processing algorithms, Image IQ (www.Image-IQ.com) can develop robust, automated analysis solutions tailored to a specific application, acquisition technique and staining method that are thoroughly validated with appropriate positive and negative controls.

These solutions provide flexible, user-defined morphometric/intensity outcome parameters circumventing the steep learning curves associated with commercial packages. An example of cytometric image analysis enabled by Image IQ from an FNAB of uveal melanoma is demonstrated (fig. 5). The entire analysis procedure did not require user interaction, output data to Excel for every image analyzed, and generated a pseudocolored representation of the segmented structures for visual validation.

Conclusions

For the foreseeable future, ophthalmic FNAB samples will continue to be evaluated in the traditional methods by an experienced cytopathologist. Cost is perhaps the only thing holding back further development and integration of these newer technologies into widespread clinical usage taking them out of the realm of research applications. With reduction in the costs, further enhancement in the scanning technology, and constantly improving pattern recognition software, the pros will far outweigh the contras of digital cytology. Advances in technology will continue to shape how cytological evaluations are performed with increasing automation and incorporation of subjective criteria. It is expected that shift toward digital technology will not only improve the diagnostic certainty of interpretations but will also facilitate education and training of future cytopathologists.

References

1 Fastenberg DM, Finger PT, Chess Q, Koizumi JH, Packer S: Vitrectomy retinotomy aspiration biopsy of choroidal tumors. Am J Ophthalmol 1990;110:361–365.

2 Arbour JD, Mukai S: Biopsy of the retina and the choroid. Int Ophthalmol Clin 1999;39:213–222.

3 Foulds WS: The uses and limitations of intraocular biopsy. Eye (Lond) 1992;6:11–27.

4 Bechrakis NE, Foerster MH, Bornfeld N: Biopsy in indeterminate intraocular tumors. Ophthalmology 2002;109:235–242.

5 Kvanta A, Seregard S, Kopp ED, All-Ericsson C, Landau I, Berglin L: Choroidal biopsies for intraocular tumors of indeterminate origin. Am J Ophthalmol 2005;140:1002–1006.

6 Sen J, Groenewald C, Hiscott PS, Smith PA, Damato BE: Transretinal choroidal tumor biopsy with a 25-gauge vitrector. Ophthalmology 2006; 113:1028–1031.

7 Char DH: Intraocular biopsy; in Singh AD, Damato BE, Pe'er J, Murphree AL, Perry JD (eds): Clinical Ophthalmic Oncology. Philadelphia, Saunders-Elsevier, 2007, pp 334–340.

8 Shields JA, Shields CL, Ehya H, Eagle RC Jr, De Potter P: Fine-needle aspiration biopsy of suspected intraocular tumors. Int Ophthalmol Clin 1993;33:77–82.

9 Young TA, Burgess BL, Rao NP, Glasgow BJ, Straatsma BR: Transscleral fine-needle aspiration biopsy of macular choroidal melanoma. Am J Ophthalmol 2008;145:297–302.

10 Singh AD, Pelayes D, Zarate JO, Biscotti CV: FNAB of uveal melanoma with a graded prototype needle. ARVO Meet Abstr 2011;52:3270.

11 Torres V, Triozzi P, Eng C, et al: Circulating tumor cells in uveal melanoma. Future Oncol 2011; 7:101–109.

12 Tang F, Lao K, Surani MA: Development and applications of single-cell transcriptome analysis. Nat Methods 2011;8(suppl):S6–S11.

13 Ulmer A, Beutel J, Susskind D, et al: Visualization of circulating melanoma cells in peripheral blood of patients with primary uveal melanoma. Clin Cancer Res 2008;14:4469–4474.

14 Ulmer A, Schmidt-Kittler O, Fischer J, et al: Immunomagnetic enrichment, genomic characterization, and prognostic impact of circulating melanoma cells. Clin Cancer Res 2004;10:531–537.

15 Augsburger JJ, Shields JA, Folberg R, Lang W, O'Hara BJ, Claricci JD: Fine needle aspiration biopsy in the diagnosis of intraocular cancer. cytologic-histologic correlations. Ophthalmology 1985;92:39–49.

16 Shields JA, Shields CL, Ehya H, Eagle RC Jr, De Potter P: Fine-needle aspiration biopsy of suspected intraocular tumors: the 1992 Urwick lecture. Ophthalmology 1993;100:1677–1684.

17 Varadhachary GR, Spector Y, Abbruzzese JL, et al: Prospective gene signature study using microRNA to identify the tissue of origin in patients with carcinoma of unknown primary (CUP). Clin Cancer Res 2011;17:4063–4070.

18 Ferracin M, Pedriali M, Veronese A, et al: MicroRNA profiling for the identification of cancers with unknown primary tissue-of-origin. J Pathol 2011;225:43–53.

19 Char DH, Ljung BM, Deschenes J, Miller TR: Intraocular lymphoma: immunological and cytological analysis. Br J Ophthalmol 1988;72:905–911.

20 Kocjan G: Best practice No 185: cytological and molecular diagnosis of lymphoma. J Clin Pathol 2005;58:561–567.

21 Davis JL, Solomon D, Nussenblatt RB, Palestine AG, Chan CC: Immunocytochemical staining of vitreous cells: indications, techniques, and results. Ophthalmology 1992;99:250–256.

22 Davis JL, Viciana AL, Ruiz P: Diagnosis of intraocular lymphoma by flow cytometry. Am J Ophthalmol 1997;124:362–372.

23 Farkas T, Harbour JW, Davila RM: Cytologic diagnosis of intraocular lymphoma in vitreous aspirates. Acta Cytol 2004;48:487–491.

24 Sweetenham JW: Molecular signatures in the diagnosis and management of diffuse large B-cell lymphoma. Curr Opin Hematol 2011;18:288–292.

25 Sisley K, Rennie IG, Parsons MA, et al: Abnormalities of chromosomes 3 and 8 in posterior uveal melanoma correlate with prognosis. Genes Chromosomes Cancer 1997;19:22–28.

26 Onken MD, Worley LA, Tuscan MD, Harbour JW: An accurate, clinically feasible multi-gene expression assay for predicting metastasis in uveal melanoma. J Mol Diagn 2010;12:461–468.

27 O'Brien MJ, Takahashi M, Brugal G, et al: Digital imagery/telecytology: International Academy of Cytology Task Force summary. Diagnostic cytology towards the 21st century: an international expert conference and tutorial. Acta Cytol 1998; 42:148–164.

28 Wilbur DC: Digital cytology: current state of the art and prospects for the future. Acta Cytol 2011; 55:227–238.

29 Giansanti D, Grigioni M, D'Avenio G, et al: Virtual microscopy and digital cytology: state of the art. Ann Ist Super Sanita 2010;46:115–122.

30 Hanselmann M, Kothe U, Kirchner M, et al: Toward digital staining using imaging mass spectrometry and random forests. J Proteome Res 2009;8:3558–3567.

31 Pham NA, Morrison A, Schwock J, et al: Quantitative image analysis of immunohistochemical stains using a CMYK color model. Diagn Pathol 2007;2:8.

32 Marganski WA, El-Sirgany Costa V, Kilpatrick MW, Tafas T, Yim J, Matthews M: Digitized microscopy in the diagnosis of bladder cancer: analysis of >3,000 cases during a 7-month period. Cancer Cytopathol 2011, E-pub ahead of print.

33 Kerr SE, Bellizzi AM, Stelow EB, Frierson HF Jr, Policarpio-Nicolas ML: Initial assessment of fine-needle aspiration specimens by telepathology: validation for use in pathology resident-faculty consultations. Am J Clin Pathol 2008;130: 409–413.

34 Heimann A, Maini G, Hwang S, Shroyer KR, Singh M. Use of telecytology for the immediate assessment of CT guided and endoscopic FNA cytology: diagnostic accuracy, advantages, and pitfalls. Diagn Cytopathol 2010, E-pub ahead of print.

35 Tsuchihashi Y. Expanding application of digital pathology in Japan – from education, telepathology to autodiagnosis. Diagn Pathol 2011;6(suppl 1):S19.

36 Pinco J, Goulart RA, Otis CN, Garb J, Pantanowitz L: Impact of digital image manipulation in cytology. Arch Pathol Lab Med 2009;133: 57–61.

37 Doyle S, Rodriguez C, Madabhushi A, Tomaszeweski J, Feldman M: Detecting prostatic adenocarcinoma from digitized histology using a multi-scale hierarchical classification approach. Conf Proc IEEE Eng Med Biol Soc 2006;1:4759–4762.

38 Gilbert DF, Meinhof T, Pepperkok R, Runz H: DetecTiff: a novel image analysis routine for high-content screening microscopy. J Biomol Screen 2009;14:944–955.

Arun D. Singh, MD, Professor of Ophthalmology
Director, Department of Ophthalmic Oncology, Cole Eye Institute, Cleveland Clinic Foundation
Euclid Avenue
Cleveland, OH 44195 (USA)
Tel. +1 216 445 9479, E-Mail singha@ccf.org

Author Index

Subject Index